Understanding Addiction

Understanding Addiction

Edited by Sidney Forsyth

hayle medical

New York

Hayle Medical,
750 Third Avenue, 9th Floor,
New York, NY 10017, USA

Visit us on the World Wide Web at:
www.haylemedical.com

ISBN: 978-1-63241-522-6

The publisher's policy is to use permanent paper from mills that operate a sustainable forestry policy. Furthermore, the publisher ensures that the text paper and cover boards used have met acceptable environmental accreditation standards.

Printed in China.

Cataloging-in-Publication Data

Understanding addiction / edited by Sidney Forsyth.
p. cm.
Includes bibliographical references and index.
ISBN 978-1-63241-522-6
1. Compulsive behavior. 2. Substance abuse. I. Forsyth, Sidney.

RC533 .U53 2018
616.852 27--dc23

Table of Contents

Preface .... **VII**

Chapter 1 **A Brief Introduction to Addiction** **1**

a. Addiction 1
b. Addictive Behavior 14

Chapter 2 **Diverse Types of Addiction** **17**

a. Cocaine Dependence 17
b. Nicotine 19
c. Alcoholism 31
d. Amphetamine 52
e. Food Addiction 72
f. Gambling Addiction 76
g. Sexual Addiction 84
h. Behavioral Addiction 90
i. Shopping Addiction 93

Chapter 3 **Substance Abuse and Disorders** **101**

a. Substance Abuse 101
b. Substance Use Disorder 130
c. Opioid Use Disorder 138
d. Amphetamine Dependence 149

Chapter 4 **Understanding Addiction Psychology and Psychiatry** **151**

a. Addiction Psychology 151
b. Addiction Vulnerability 160
c. Addiction Psychiatry 163

Chapter 5 **Treatment for Addiction** **167**

a. Addiction Medicine 167
b. Drug Rehabilitation 182
c. Nicotine Replacement Therapy 200

d. Varenicline 204
e. Coding (Therapy) 207
f. Contingency Management 208
g. Community Reinforcement Approach and Family Training 210

Permissions

Index

Preface

Addiction is a type of brain disorder which results in compulsive engagement of stimuli, even when the subject is aware of its negative consequences. The behavior is triggered if the body does not get the reward. The most common sources of addiction are opium, nicotine, alcohol, sex, food, cocaine, amphetamine, or gambling. The treatment generally includes medication and behavioral therapy. The book aims to shed light on some of the unexplored aspects of addiction. It provides deep insights about the concepts, theories, and treatment of these addictions. This textbook presents the complex subject of addiction in the most comprehensible and easy to understand language. This book, with its detailed analysis and data, will prove immensely beneficial to professionals and students involved in this area.

A detailed account of the significant topics covered in this book is provided below:

Chapter 1- Addiction is a disorder of the brain which causes an uncontrollable urge to an addictive stimuli like cocaine, gambling, sex or morphine. It is caused by epigenetic and transgenic problems in the brain's reward system. The chapter on addiction offers an insightful focus, keeping in mind the complex subject matter.

Chapter 2- The different types of addiction discussed in this section are cocaine dependence, nicotine, food addiction, amphetamine, alcoholism, sexual addiction, behavioral addiction and shopping addiction. Cocaine dependence is the dependence one feels towards drugs. It has withdrawal symptoms such as depression, anxiety, dysphoria and compulsive cravings. The topics discussed in the chapter are of great importance to broaden the existing knowledge on types of addiction.

Chapter 3- Dependency on drugs that alter perception and consciousness of users is substance abuse. Mood changes, problems at work or school, change in behavior or changing in eating habits are some symptoms of substance abuse. Substance use disorder, opioid use disorder and amphetamine dependence are some topics explained in the following chapter.

Chapter 4- Addiction psychology consists of two parts, clinical and abnormal psychology. The two models of addicts considered by professional are diseases model of addiction and the choice model of addiction. Cognitive therapy and behaviorism are used to combat addiction. The chapter serves as a source to understand addiction psychology and psychiatry.

Chapter 5- Addiction can be treated by therapy, counseling or by medication. Addiction medicine is the treatment given for addiction. Drug rehabilitation, nicotine replacement therapy, coding, contingency management and community reinforcement approach and family training are some diagnosis and treatments discussed in the following section. Addiction is best understood in confluence with the major topics listed in the following chapter.

I would like to make a special mention of my publisher who considered me worthy of this opportunity and also supported me throughout the process. I would also like to thank the editing team at the back-end who extended their help whenever required.

Editor

1

A Brief Introduction to Addiction

Addiction is a disorder of the brain which causes an uncontrollable urge to an addictive stimuli like cocaine, gambling, sex or morphine. It is caused by epigenetic and transgenic problems in the brain's reward system. The chapter on addiction offers an insightful focus, keeping in mind the complex subject matter.

Addiction

Addiction is a brain disorder characterized by compulsive engagement in rewarding stimuli, despite adverse consequences. Despite the involvement of a number of psychosocial factors, a biological process – one which is induced by repeated exposure to an addictive stimulus – is the core pathology that drives the development and maintenance of an addiction. The two properties that characterize all addictive stimuli are that they are reinforcing (i.e., they increase the likelihood that a person will seek repeated exposure to them) and intrinsically rewarding (i.e., they are perceived as being inherently positive, desirable, and pleasurable).

Addiction is a disorder of the brain's reward system which arises through transcriptional and epigenetic mechanisms and occurs over time from chronically high levels of exposure to an addictive stimulus (e.g., morphine, cocaine, sexual intercourse, gambling, etc.). ΔFosB, a gene transcription factor, is a critical component and common factor in the development of virtually all forms of behavioral and drug addictions. Two decades of research into ΔFosB's role in addiction have demonstrated that addiction arises, and the associated compulsive behavior intensifies or attenuates, along with the overexpression of ΔFosB in the D1-type medium spiny neurons of the nucleus accumbens. Due to the causal relationship between ΔFosB expression and addictions, it is used preclinically as an addiction biomarker. ΔFosB expression in these neurons directly and positively regulates drug self-administration and reward sensitization through positive reinforcement, while decreasing sensitivity to aversion.

As described by two groups of researchers, addiction exacts an "astoundingly high financial and human toll" on individuals and society as a whole through the direct adverse effects of drugs, associated healthcare costs, long-term complications (e.g., lung cancer with smoking tobacco, liver cirrhosis with drinking alcohol, or meth mouth from intravenous methamphetamine), the functional consequences of altered neural plasticity in the brain, and the consequent loss of productivity. Classic hallmarks of addiction include impaired control over substances or behavior, preoccupation with substance or behavior, and continued use despite consequences. Habits and patterns associated with addiction are typically characterized by immediate gratification (short-term reward), coupled with delayed deleterious effects (long-term costs).

Examples of drug and behavioral addictions include: alcoholism, amphetamine addiction, cocaine addiction, nicotine addiction, opiate addiction, food addiction, gambling addiction, and sexual addiction. The only behavioral addiction recognized by the DSM-5 is gambling addiction. The term *addiction* is misused frequently to refer to other compulsive behaviors or disorders, particularly *dependence*, in news media. An important distinction between drug addiction and dependence is that drug dependence is a disorder in which cessation of drug use results in an unpleasant state of withdrawal, which can lead to further drug use. Addiction is the compulsive use of a substance or performance of a behavior that is independent of withdrawal.

Neuropsychology

Cognitive control and stimulus control, which is associated with operant and classical conditioning, represent opposite processes (i.e., internal vs external or environmental, respectively) that compete over the control of an individual's elicited behaviors. Cognitive control, and particularly inhibitory control over behavior, is impaired in both addiction and attention deficit hyperactivity disorder. Stimulus-driven behavioral responses (i.e., stimulus control) that are associated with a particular rewarding stimulus tend to dominate one's behavior in an addiction.

Behavioral Addiction

The term *behavioral addiction* correctly refers to a compulsion to engage in a natural reward – which is a behavior that is inherently rewarding (i.e., desirable or appealing) – despite adverse consequences. Preclinical evidence has demonstrated that marked increases in the expression of ΔFosB through repetitive and excessive exposure to a natural reward induces the same behavioral effects and neuroplasticity as occurs in a drug addiction.

Reviews of both clinical research in humans and preclinical studies involving ΔFosB have identified compulsive sexual activity – specifically, any form of sexual intercourse – as an addiction (i.e., sexual addiction). Moreover, reward cross-sensitization between amphetamine and sexual activity, a property in which exposure to one increases in the desire for both, has been shown to occur preclinically and clinically as a dopamine dysregulation syndrome; ΔFosB expression is required for this cross-sensitization effect, which intensifies with the level of ΔFosB expression.

Reviews of preclinical studies indicate that long-term frequent and excessive consumption of high fat or sugar foods can produce an addiction (food addiction).

Gambling is a natural reward which is associated with compulsive behavior and for which clinical diagnostic manuals, namely the DSM-5, have identified diagnostic criteria for an "addiction". There is evidence from functional neuroimaging that gambling activates the reward system and the mesolimbic pathway in particular. Similarly, shopping and playing videogames are associated with compulsive behaviors in humans and have also been shown to activate the mesolimbic pathway and other parts of the reward system. Based upon this evidence, gambling addiction, video game addiction and shopping addiction are classified accordingly.

Risk Factors

There are a range of genetic and environmental risk factors for developing an addiction that vary across the population. Roughly half of an individual's risk for developing an addiction is derived from genetics, while the other half is derived from the environment. However, even in individuals with a relatively low genetic loading, exposure to sufficiently high doses of an addictive drug for a long period of time (e.g., weeks–months) can result in an addiction. In other words, anyone can become an addict under the right circumstances.

Age

Adolescence represents a period of unique vulnerability for developing addiction. Not only are adolescents more likely to initiate and maintain drug use, but once addicted they are more resistant to treatment and more liable to relapse. Statistics have shown that those who start to drink alcohol at a younger age are more likely to become dependent later on. About 33% of the population tasted their first alcohol between the ages of 15 and 17, while 18% experienced it prior to this. As for alcohol abuse or dependence, the numbers start off high with those who first drank before they were 12 and then drop off after that. For example, 16% of alcoholics began drinking prior to turning 12 years old, while only 9% first touched alcohol between 15 and 17. This percentage is even lower, at 2.6%, for those who first started the habit after they were 21.

Genetic Factors

It has long been established that genetic factors along with social and psychological factors are contributors to addiction. A common theory along these lines is the self-medication hypothesis. Epidemiological studies estimate that genetic factors account for 40–60% of the risk factors for alcoholism. Similar rates of heritability for other types of drug addiction have been indicated by other studies. Knestler hypothesized in 1964 that a gene or group of genes might contribute to predisposition to addiction in several ways. For example, altered levels of a normal protein due to environmental factors could then change the structure or functioning of specific brain neurons during development. These altered brain neurons could change the susceptibility of an individual to an initial drug use experience. In support of this hypothesis, animal studies have shown that environmental factors such as stress can affect an animal's genotype.

Overall, the data implicating specific genes in the development of drug addiction is mixed for most genes. One reason for this may be that the case is due to a focus of current research on common variants. Many addiction studies focus on common variants with an allele frequency of greater than 5% in the general population, however when associated with disease, these only confer a small amount of additional risk with an odds ratio of 1.1–1.3 percent. On the other hand, the rare variant hypothesis states that genes with low frequencies in the population (<1%) confer much greater additional risk in the development of disease.

Genome-wide association studies (GWAS) are a recently developed research method which are used to examine genetic associations with dependence, addiction, and drug use. These studies employ an unbiased approach to finding genetic associations with specific phenotypes and give equal weight to all regions of DNA, including those with no ostensible relationship to drug metabolism or response. These studies rarely identify genes from proteins previously described via animal knockout models and candidate gene analysis. Instead, large percentages of genes involved in processes such as cell adhesion are commonly identified. This is not to say that previous findings, or the GWAS findings, are erroneous. The important effects of endophenotypes are typically not capable of being captured by these methods. Furthermore, genes identified in GWAS for drug addiction may be involved either in adjusting brain behavior prior to drug experiences, subsequent to them, or both.

Environmental Factors

Adverse childhood experiences (ACEs) are various forms of maltreatment and household dysfunction experienced in childhood. The Adverse Childhood Experiences Study by the Centers for Disease Control and Prevention has shown a strong dose–response relationship between ACEs and numerous health, social, and behavioral problems throughout a person's lifespan, including those associated with substance abuse. Children's neurological development can be disrupted when they are chronically exposed to stressful events such as physical, emotional, or sexual abuse, physical or emotional neglect, witnessing violence in the household, or a parent being incarcerated or suffering from a mental illness. As a result, the child's cognitive functioning or ability to cope with negative or disruptive emotions may be impaired. Over time, the child may adopt substance use as a coping mechanism, particularly during adolescence.

The National Institute on Drug Abuse cites lack of parental supervision, the prevalence of peer substance use, drug availability, and poverty as risk factors for substance use development.

Psychological Factors

Individuals with comorbid (i.e., co-occurring) mental health disorders such as depression, anxiety, attention-deficit/hyperactivity disorder (ADHD) or post-traumatic stress disorder are more likely to develop substance use disorders.

The National Institute on Drug Abuse cites early aggressive behavior as a risk factor for substance use development.

Transgenerational Epigenetic Inheritance

Epigenetic genes and their products (e.g., proteins) are the key components through which environmental influences can affect the genes of an individual; they also serve as the mechanism responsible for the transgenerational epigenetic inheritance of behavioral phenotypes, a phenomenon in which environmental influences on the genes of a parent can affect the associated traits and behavioral phenotypes of their offspring (e.g., behavioral responses to certain environmental stimuli). In addiction, epigenetic mechanisms play a central role in the pathophysiology of the disease; it has been noted that some of the alterations to the epigenome which arise through chronic exposure to addictive stimuli during an addiction can be transmitted across generations, in turn affecting the behavior of one's children (e.g., the child's behavioral responses to addictive drugs and natural rewards). More research is needed to determine the specific epigenetic mechanisms and the nature of heritable behavioral phenotypes that arise from addictions in humans. Based upon preclinical evidence with lab animals, the addiction-related behavioral phenotypes that are transmitted across generations may serve to increase or decrease the child's risk of developing an addiction.

Mechanisms

Chronic addictive drug use causes alterations in gene expression in the mesocorticolimbic projection. The most important transcription factors that produce these alterations are ΔFosB, cAMP response element binding protein (CREB), and nuclear factor kappa B (NF-κB). ΔFosB is the most significant biomolecular mechanism in addiction because the overexpression of ΔFosB in the D1-type medium spiny neurons in the nucleus accumbens is necessary and sufficient for many of the neural adaptations and behavioral effects (e.g., expression-dependent increases in drug self-administration and reward sensitization) seen in drug addiction. ΔFosB expression in nucleus accumbens D1-type medium spiny neurons directly and positively regulates drug self-administration and reward sensitization through positive reinforcement while decreasing sensitivity to aversion. Specific drug addictions in which ΔFosB has been implicated in addictions to alcohol, amphetamine, cannabinoids, cocaine, methylphenidate, nicotine, phenylcyclidine, propofol, opiates, and substituted amphetamines, among others. ΔJunD, a transcription factor, and G9a, a histone methyltransferase, both oppose the function of

ΔFosB and inhibit increases in its expression. Increases in nucleus accumbens ΔJunD expression (via viral vector-mediated gene transfer) or G9a expression (via pharmacological means) reduces, or with a large increase can even block, many of the neural and behavioral alterations seen in chronic drug abuse (i.e., the alterations mediated by ΔFosB).

ΔFosB also plays an important role in regulating behavioral responses to natural rewards, such as palatable food, sex, and exercise. Natural rewards, like drugs of abuse, induce gene expression of ΔFosB in the nucleus accumbens, and chronic acquisition of these rewards can result in a similar pathological addictive state through ΔFosB overexpression. Consequently, ΔFosB is the key transcription factor involved in addictions to natural rewards (i.e., behavioral addictions) as well; in particular, ΔFosB in the nucleus accumbens is critical for the reinforcing effects of sexual reward. Research on the interaction between natural and drug rewards suggests that dopaminergic psychostimulants (e.g., amphetamine) and sexual behavior act on similar biomolecular mechanisms to induce ΔFosB in the nucleus accumbens and possess bidirectional cross-sensitization effects that are mediated through ΔFosB. This phenomenon is notable since, in humans, a dopamine dysregulation syndrome, characterized by drug-induced compulsive engagement in natural rewards (specifically, sexual activity, shopping, and gambling), has also been observed in some individuals taking dopaminergic medications.

ΔFosB inhibitors (drugs or treatments that oppose its action) may be an effective treatment for addiction and addictive disorders.

The release of dopamine in the nucleus accumbens plays a role in the reinforcing qualities of many forms of stimuli, including naturally reinforcing stimuli like palatable food and sex. Altered dopamine neurotransmission is frequently observed following the development of an addictive state. In humans and lab animals that have developed an addiction, alterations in dopamine or opioid neurotransmission in the nucleus accumbens and other parts of the striatum are evident. Studies have found that use of certain drugs (e.g., cocaine) affect cholinergic neurons that innervate the reward system, in turn affecting dopamine signaling in this region.

Reward System

Mesocorticolimbic Pathway

In the images below the top image depicts, the initial effects of high dose exposure to an addictive drug on gene expression in the nucleus accumbens for various genes in the Fos family. While the bottom image illustrates the progressive increase in ΔFosB expression in the nucleus accumbens following repeated twice daily drug binges, where these phosphorylated (35–37 kD) ΔFosB isoforms persist in the D1-type medium spiny neurons of the nucleus accumbens for up to 2 months.

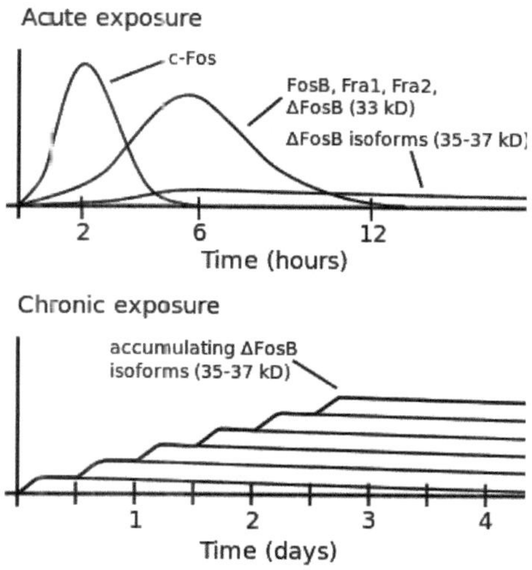

ΔFosB accumulation from excessive drug use

Understanding the pathways in which drugs act and how drugs can alter those pathways is key when examining the biological basis of drug addiction. The reward pathway, known as the mesolimbic pathway, or its extension, the mesocorticolimbic pathway, is characterized by the interaction of several areas of the brain.

- The projections from the ventral tegmental area (VTA) are a network of dopaminergic neurons with co-localized postsynaptic glutamate receptors (AMPAR and NMDAR). These cells respond when stimuli indicative of a reward are present. The VTA supports learning and sensitization development and releases DA into the forebrain. These neurons also project and release DA into the nucleus accumbens, through the mesolimbic pathway. Virtually all drugs causing drug addiction increase the dopamine release in the mesolimbic pathway, in addition to their specific effects.

- The nucleus accumbens (NAcc) is one output of the VTA projections. The nucleus accumbens itself consists mainly of GABAergic medium spiny neurons (MSNs). The NAcc is associated with acquiring and eliciting conditioned behaviors, and is involved in the increased sensitivity to drugs as addiction progresses. Overexpression of ΔFosB in the nucleus accumbens is a necessary common factor in essentially all known forms of addiction; ΔFosB is a strong positive modulator of positively reinforced behaviors.

- The prefrontal cortex, including the anterior cingulate and orbitofrontal cortices, is another VTA output in the mesocorticolimbic pathway; it is important for the integration of information which helps determine whether a behavior will be elicited. It is also critical for forming associations between the rewarding experience of drug use and cues in the environment. Importantly, these cues are strong mediators of drug-seeking behavior and can trigger relapse even after months or years of abstinence.

Other brain structures that are involved in addiction include:

- The basolateral amygdala projects into the NAcc and is thought to also be important for motivation.
- The hippocampus is involved in drug addiction, because of its role in learning and memory. Much of this evidence stems from investigations showing that manipulating cells in the hippocampus alters dopamine levels in NAcc and firing rates of VTA dopaminergic cells.

Role of Dopamine and Glutamate

Dopamine is the primary neurotransmitter of the reward system in the brain. It plays a role in regulating movement, emotion, cognition, motivation, and feelings of pleasure. Natural rewards, like eating, as well as recreational drug use cause a release of dopamine, and are associated with the reinforcing nature of these stimuli. Nearly all addictive drugs, directly or indirectly, act upon the brain's reward system by heightening dopaminergic activity.

Excessive intake of many types of addictive drugs results in repeated release of high amounts of dopamine, which in turn affects the reward pathway directly through heightened dopamine receptor activation. Prolonged and abnormally high levels of dopamine in the synaptic cleft can induce receptor downregulation in the neural pathway. Downregulation of mesolimbic dopamine receptors can result in a decrease in the sensitivity to natural reinforcers.

Drug seeking behavior is induced by glutamatergic projections from the prefrontal cortex to the nucleus accumbens. This idea is supported with data from experiments showing that drug seeking behavior can be prevented following the inhibition of AMPA glutamate receptors and glutamate release in the nucleus accumbens.

Reward Sensitization

Reward sensitization is a process that causes an increase in the amount of reward (specifically, incentive salience) that is assigned by the brain to a rewarding stimulus (e.g., a drug). In simple terms, when reward sensitization to a specific stimulus (e.g., a drug) occurs, an individual's "wanting" or desire for the stimulus itself and its associated cues increases. Reward sensitization normally occurs following chronically high levels of exposure to the stimulus. ΔFosB (DeltaFosB) expression in D1-type medium spiny neurons in the nucleus accumbens has been shown to directly and positively regulate reward sensitization involving drugs and natural rewards.

"Cue-induced wanting" or "cue-triggered wanting", a form of craving that occurs in addiction, is responsible for the majority of compulsive behavior that addicts exhibit. These cues create overwhelming short-term urges to engage an addictive stimulus by acting as conditioned reinforcers for the addictive stimulus (a primary reinforcer) that are assigned pathologically high levels of incentive salience ("want").

Neural and Behavioral Effects of Validated ΔFosB Transcriptional Targets			
Target gene	**Target expression**	**Neural effects**	**Behavioral effects**
c-Fos	↓	• Molecular switch enabling the chronic induction of ΔFosB	–
dynorphin	↓	• Downregulation of κ-opioid feedback loop	• Increased drug reward
NF-κB	↑	• Expansion of NAcc dendritic processes • NF-κB inflammatory response in the NAcc • NF-κB inflammatory response in the CP	• Increased drug reward • Increased drug reward • Locomotor sensitization
GluR2	↑	• Decreased sensitivity to glutamate	• Increased drug reward
Cdk5	↑	• GluR1 synaptic protein phosphorylation • Expansion of NAcc dendritic processes	• Decreased drug reward (net effect)

Research on the interaction between natural and drug rewards suggests that dopaminergic psychostimulants (e.g., amphetamine) and sexual behavior act on similar biomolecular mechanisms to induce ΔFosB in the nucleus accumbens and possess a bidirectional reward cross-sensitization effect that is mediated through ΔFosB.

In contrast to ΔFosB's reward-sensitizing effect, CREB transcriptional activity decreases user's sensitivity to the rewarding effects of the substance. CREB transcription in the nucleus accumbens is implicated in psychological dependence and symptoms involving a lack of pleasure or motivation during drug withdrawal.

The set of proteins known as "regulators of G protein signaling" (RGS), particularly RGS4 and RGS9-2, have been implicated in modulating some forms of opioid sensitization, including reward sensitization.

Diagnosis

The 5th edition of the Diagnostic and Statistical Manual of Mental Disorders (DSM-5) uses the term "Substance Use Disorder" to refer to a spectrum of use-related conditions. The DSM-5 eliminates the terms "abuse" and "dependence" from diagnostic categories, instead using the specifiers of "mild", "moderate" and "severe" to indicate the extent of disordered use. Specifiers are determined by the number of diagnostic criteria present in a given case. The manual has never actually used the term "addiction" clinically. Currently, only drug addictions and gambling addiction are listed in the DSM-5. Past editions have used physical dependence and the associated withdrawal syndrome to identify an addictive state. Physical dependence occurs when the body has adjusted by incorporating the substance into its "normal" functioning – i.e., attains homeostasis – and therefore physical withdrawal symptoms occur upon cessation of use. Tolerance is the process by which the body continually adapts to the substance and requires increasingly larger amounts to achieve the original effects. Withdrawal refers to physical and psychological symptoms experienced when reducing or discontinuing a substance that the body has become dependent on. Symptoms of withdrawal generally include but are not limited to anxiety, irritability, intense cravings for the substance, nausea, hallucinations, headaches, cold sweats, and tremors.

Medical researchers who actively study addiction have criticized the DSM classification of addiction for being flawed and involving arbitrary diagnostic criteria. Writing in 2013, the director of the United States National Institute of Mental Health discussed the invalidity of the DSM-5's classification of mental disorders.

While DSM has been described as a "Bible" for the field, it is, at best, a dictionary, creating a set of labels and defining each. The strength of each of the editions of DSM has been "reliability" – each edition has ensured that clinicians use the same terms in the same ways. The weakness is its lack of validity. Unlike our definitions of ischemic heart disease, lymphoma, or AIDS, the DSM diagnoses are based on a consensus about clusters of clinical symptoms, not any objective laboratory measure. In the rest of medicine, this would be equivalent to creating diagnostic systems based on the nature of chest pain or the quality of fever.

Most recently, though, the NIH acknowledged advances in identifying biomarkers, noting they outperform traditional phenomenological categories in identifying types of psychosis. As a diagnostic biomarker, ΔFosB expression could be used to diagnose an addiction in humans, but this would require a brain biopsy and therefore isn't used in clinical practice.

Treatment

According to a review, "in order to be effective, all pharmacological or biologically based treatments for addiction need to be integrated into other established forms of addiction rehabilitation, such as cognitive behavioral therapy, individual and group psychotherapy, behavior-modification strategies, twelve-step programs, and residential treatment facilities."

Behavioral Therapy

A meta-analytic review on the efficacy of various behavioral therapies for treating drug and behavioral addictions found that cognitive behavioral therapy (e.g., relapse prevention and contingency management), motivational interviewing, and a community reinforcement approach were effective interventions with moderate effect sizes. Preclinical research using a rodent model of cue exposure therapy (CET) show that this type of treatment is more effective in adults compared to adolescents, however that adolescent outcomes can be improved by acute treatment at the time of (CET) with a dopamine 2 receptor agonist.

Clinical and preclinical evidence indicate that consistent aerobic exercise, especially endurance exercise (e.g., marathon running), actually prevents the development of certain drug addictions and is an effective adjunct treatment for drug addiction, and for psychostimulant addiction in particular. Consistent aerobic exercise magnitude-dependently (i.e., by duration and intensity) reduces drug addiction risk, which appears to occur through the reversal of drug induced addiction-related neuroplasticity. One review noted that exercise may prevent the development of drug addiction by altering ΔFosB or c-Fos immunoreactivity in the striatum or other parts of the reward system. Aerobic exercise decreases drug self-administration, reduces the likelihood of relapse, and induces opposite effects on striatal dopamine receptor D_2 (DRD2) signaling (increased DRD2 density) to those induced by addictions to several drug classes (decreased DRD2 density). Consequently, consistent aerobic exercise may lead to better treatment outcomes when used as an adjunct treatment for drug addiction.

Medication

Alcohol Addiction

Alcohol, like opioids, can induce a severe state of physical dependence and produce withdrawal symptoms such as delirium tremens. Because of this, treatment for alcohol addiction usually involves a combined approach dealing with dependence and addiction simultaneously.

Pharmacological treatments for alcohol addiction include drugs like naltrexone (opioid antagonist), disulfiram, acamprosate, and topiramate. Rather than substituting for alcohol, these drugs are intended to affect the desire to drink, either by directly reducing cravings as with acamprosate and topiramate, or by producing unpleasant effects when alcohol is consumed, as with disulfiram. These drugs can be effective if treatment is maintained, but compliance can be an issue as alcoholic patients often forget to take their medication, or discontinue use because of excessive side effects. According to a Cochrane Collaboration review, the opioid antagonist naltrexone has been shown to be an effective treatment for alcholism, with the effects lasting three to twelve months after the end of treatment.

Behavioral Addictions

Behavioral addiction is a treatable condition. Treatment options include psychotherapy and psychopharmacotherapy (i.e., medications) or a combination of both. Cognitive behavioral therapy (CBT) is the most common form of psychotherapy used in treating behavioral addictions; it focuses on identifying patterns that trigger compulsive behavior and making lifestyle changes to promote healthier behaviors. Currently, there are no medications approved for treatment of behavioral addictions in general, but some medications used for treatment of drug addiction may also be beneficial with specific behavioral addictions.

Cannabinoid Addiction

As of 2010, there are no effective pharmacological interventions for cannabinoid addiction. A 2013 review on cannabinoid addiction noted that the development of CB1 receptor agonists that have reduced interaction with β-arrestin 2 signaling might be therapeutically useful.

Nicotine Addiction

Another area in which drug treatment has been widely used is in the treatment of nicotine addiction, which usually involves the use of nicotine replacement therapy, nicotinic receptor antagonists, or nicotinic receptor partial agonists. Examples of drugs that act on nicotinic receptors and have been used for treating nicotine addiction include antagonists like bupropion and the partial agonist varenicline.

Opioid Addiction

Opioids cause physical dependence, and treatment typically addresses both dependence and addiction.

Physical dependence is treated using replacement drugs such as suboxone or subutex (both containing the active ingredients buprenorphine) and methadone. Although these drugs perpetuate physical dependence, the goal of opiate maintenance is to provide a measure of control over both pain and cravings. Use of replacement drugs increases the patient's ability to function normally and eliminates the negative consequences of obtaining controlled substances illicitly. Once a prescribed dosage is stabilized, treatment enters maintenance or tapering phases. In the United States, opiate replacement therapy is tightly regulated in methadone clinics and under the DATA 2000 legislation. In some countries, other opioid derivatives such as levomethadyl acetate, dihydrocodeine, dihydroetorphine and even heroin are used as substitute drugs for illegal street opiates, with different prescriptions being given depending on the needs of the individual patient. Baclofen has led to successful reductions of cravings for stimulants, alcohol, and opioids, and also alleviates alcohol withdrawal syndrome. Many patients have stated they "became indifferent to alcohol" or "indifferent to cocaine" overnight after starting baclofen therapy.

Psychostimulant Addiction

As of May 2014, there is no effective pharmacotherapy for any form of psychostimulant addiction. Reviews from 2015 and 2016 indicated that TAAR1-selective agonists have significant therapeutic potential as a treatment for psychostimulant addictions; however, as of February 2016, the only compounds which are known to function as TAAR1-selective agonists are experimental drugs.

Research

Research indicates that vaccines which utilize anti-drug monoclonal antibodies can mitigate drug-induced positive reinforcement by preventing the drug from moving across the blood–brain barrier; however, current vaccine-based therapies are only effective in a relatively small subset of individuals. As of November 2015, vaccine-based therapies are being tested in human clinical trials as a treatment for addiction and preventative measure against drug overdoses involving nicotine, cocaine, and methamphetamine.

Since addiction involves abnormalities in glutamate and GABAergic neurotransmission, receptors associated with these neurotransmitters (e.g., AMPA receptors, NMDA receptors, and GABAB receptors) are potential therapeutic targets for addictions. N-acetylcysteine, which affects metabotropic glutamate receptors and NMDA receptors, has shown some benefit in preclinical and clinical studies involving addictions to cocaine, heroin, and cannabinoids. It may also be useful as an adjunct therapy for addictions to amphetamine-type stimulants, but more clinical research is required.

Current medical reviews of research involving lab animals have identified a drug class – class I histone deacetylase inhibitors – that indirectly inhibits the function and further increases in the expression of accumbal ΔFosB by inducing G9a expression in the nucleus accumbens after prolonged use. These reviews and subsequent preliminary evidence which used oral administration or intraperitoneal administration of the sodium salt of butyric acid or other class I HDAC inhibitors for an extended period indicate that these drugs have efficacy in reducing addictive behavior in lab animals that have developed addictions to ethanol, psychostimulants (i.e., amphetamine and cocaine), nicotine, and opiates; however, as of August 2015 no clinical trials involving human addicts and any HDAC class I inhibitors have been conducted to test for treatment efficacy in humans or identify an optimal dosing regimen.

Epidemiology

Due to cultural variations, the proportion of individuals who develop a drug or behavioral addiction within a specified time period (i.e., the prevalence) varies over time, by country, and across national population demographics (e.g., by age group, socioeconomic status, etc.).

Australia

The prevalence of substance abuse disorder among Australians was reported at 5.1% in 2009.

United States

Based upon representative samples of the US youth population in 2011, the lifetime prevalence of addictions to alcohol and illicit drugs has been estimated to be approximately 8% and 2–3% respectively. Based upon representative samples of US adult population in 2011, the 12 month prevalence of alcohol and illicit drug addictions were estimated at roughly 12% and 2–3% respectively. The 12 month and lifetime prevalence of prescription drug addictions is currently unknown.

As of 2016, about 22 million Americans need treatment for an addiction to alcohol, nicotine, or other drugs. Only about 10%, or a little over 2 million, receive any form of treatments, and those that do generally do not receive evidence-based care. One-third of inpatient hospital costs and 20% of all deaths in the US every year are the result of untreated addictions and risky substance use. In spite of the massive overall economic cost to society, which is greater than the cost of diabetes and all forms of cancer combined, most doctors in the US lack the training to effectively address a drug addiction.

Another review listed estimates of lifetime prevalence rates for several behavioral addictions in the United States, including 1–2% for compulsive gambling, 5% for sexual addiction, 2.8% for food addiction, and 5–6% for compulsive shopping. A systematic review indicated that the time-invariant prevalence rate for sexual addiction and related compulsive sexual behavior (e.g., compulsive masturbation with or without pornography, compulsive cybersex, etc.) within the United States ranges from 3–6% of the population.

Personality Theories of Addiction

Personality theories of addiction are psychological models that associate personality traits or modes of thinking (i.e., affective states) with an individual's proclivity for developing an addiction. Models of addiction risk that have been proposed in psychology literature include an affect dysregulation model of positive and negative psychological affects, the reinforcement sensitivity theory model of impulsiveness and behavioral inhibition, and an impulsivity model of reward sensitization and impulsiveness.

Addictive Behavior

An addictive behavior is a behavior, or a stimulus related to a behavior (e.g., sex or food), that is both rewarding and reinforcing, and is associated with the development of an addiction. Addictions involving addictive behaviors are normally referred to as behavioral addictions.

Compulsion vs Addiction

Compulsions and addictions are intertwined and reward is one major distinction between an addiction and a compulsion (as it is experienced in obsessive-compulsive disorder). An addiction is, by definition, a form of compulsion, and both addictions and compulsions involve operant reinforcement; however, in addiction, the desire and motivation to use a substance or engage in a behavior arises because it is rewarding (i.e., the compulsions that occur in addiction develop through positive reinforcement). In contrast, someone who experiences a compulsion as part of obsessive-compulsive disorder may not perceive anything rewarding from acting on the compulsion. Often, it is a way of dealing with the obsessive part of the disorder, resulting in a feeling of relief (i.e., compulsions may also arise through negative reinforcement).

Deep brain stimulation to the nucleus accumbens, a region in the brain involved heavily in addiction and reinforcement learning, has proven to be an effective treatment of obsessive compulsive disorder.

References

- Catalano RF, Hawkins JD, Wells EA, Miller J, Brewer D (1990). "Evaluation of the effectiveness of adolescent drug abuse treatment, assessment of risks for relapse, and promising approaches for relapse prevention". The International Journal of the Addictions. 25 (9A-10A): 1085–140. PMID 2131328
- "AMERICAN BOARD OF MEDICAL SPECIALTIES RECOGNIZES THE NEW SUBSPECIALTY OF ADDICTION MEDICINE" (PDF). American Board of Addiction Medicine. 14 March 2016. Retrieved 3 April 2016
- Vassoler FM, Sadri-Vakili G (2014). "Mechanisms of transgenerational inheritance of addictive-like behaviors". Neuroscience. 264: 198–206. PMC 3872494. PMID 23920159. doi:10.1016/j.neuroscience.2013.07.064
- Perepletchikova F, Krystal JH, Kaufman J (November 2008). "Practitioner review: adolescent alcohol use disorders: assessment and treatment issues". Journal of Child Psychology and Psychiatry, and Allied Disciplines. 49 (11): 1131–1154. PMC 4113213. PMID 19017028. doi:10.1111/j.1469-7610.2008.01934.x
- American Psychiatric Association (2013). "Substance-Related and Addictive Disorders" (PDF). American Psychiatric Publishing. pp. 1–2. Archived from the original (PDF) on 15 August 2015. Retrieved 10 July 2015
- Nestler EJ (December 2012). "Transcriptional mechanisms of drug addiction". Clin. Psychopharmacol. Neurosci. 10 (3): 136–143. PMC 3569166. PMID 23430970. doi:10.9758/cpn.2012.10.3.136. The 35-37 kD ΔFosB
- Kalivas PW, Volkow ND (August 2005). "The neural basis of addiction: a pathology of motivation and choice". The American Journal of Psychiatry. 162 (8): 1403–13. PMID 16055761. doi:10.1176/appi.ajp.162.8.1403
- "Adverse Childhood Experiences". samhsa.gov. Rockville, Maryland, United States: Substance Abuse and Mental Health Services Administration. Retrieved 26 September 2016

- Eisch AJ, Harburg GC (2006). "Opiates, psychostimulants, and adult hippocampal neurogenesis: Insights for addiction and stem cell biology". Hippocampus. 16 (3): 271–86. PMID 16411230. doi:10.1002/hipo.20161
- Perry CJ, Zbukvic I, Kim JH, Lawrence AJ (October 2014). "Role of cues and contexts on drug-seeking behaviour". British Journal of Pharmacology. 171 (20): 4636–72. PMC 4209936. PMID 24749941. doi:10.1111/bph.12735
- "Infographic – Risk Factors of Addiction | Recovery Research Institute". www.recoveryanswers.org. Retrieved 2016-12-19
- Soyka M, Roesner S (2006). "New pharmacological approaches for the treatment of alcoholism". Expert Opin Pharmacother. 7 (17): 2341–53. PMID 17109610. doi:10.1517/14656566.7.17.2341

2

Diverse Types of Addiction

The different types of addiction discussed in this section are cocaine dependence, nicotine, food addiction, amphetamine, alcoholism, sexual addiction, behavioral addiction and shopping addiction. Cocaine dependence is the dependence one feels towards drugs. It has withdrawal symptoms such as depression, anxiety, dysphoria and compulsive cravings. The topics discussed in the chapter are of great importance to broaden the existing knowledge on types of addiction.

Cocaine Dependence

Cocaine dependence is a psychological desire to use cocaine regularly. Cocaine overdose may result in cardiovascular and brain damage, such as: constricting blood vessels in the brain, causing strokes and constricting arteries in the heart; causing heart attacks.

The use of cocaine creates euphoria and high amounts of energy. If taken in large, unsafe doses, it is possible to cause mood swings, paranoia, insomnia, psychosis, high blood pressure, a fast heart rate, panic attacks, cognitive impairments and drastic changes in personality.

The symptoms of cocaine withdrawal (also known as *comedown or crash*) range from moderate to severe: dysphoria, depression, anxiety, psychological and physical weakness, pain, and compulsive cravings.

Signs and Symptoms

Cocaine is a powerful stimulant known to make users feel energetic, happy, talkative, etc. In time, negative side effects include increased body temperature, irregular or rapid heart rate, high blood pressure, increased risk of heart attacks, strokes and even sudden death from cardiac arrest. Many habitual abusers develop a transient, manic-like condition similar to amphetamine psychosis and schizophrenia, whose symptoms include aggression, severe paranoia, restlessness, confusion and tactile hallucinations; which can include the feeling of insects under the skin (formication), also known as "coke bugs", during binges. Users of cocaine have also reported having thoughts of suicide, unusual weight loss, trouble maintaining relationships, and an unhealthy, pale appearance.

Withdrawal Symptoms

After using cocaine on a regular basis, some users will become addicted. When the drug is discontinued immediately, the user will experience what has come to be known as a "crash" along with a number of other cocaine withdrawal symptoms, including paranoia, depression, exhaustion, anxiety, itching, mood swings, irritability, fatigue, insomnia, an intense craving for more cocaine, and in some cases nausea and vomiting. Some cocaine users also report having similar symptoms to schizophrenia patients and feel that their mind is lost. Some users also report formication: a feeling of a crawling sensation on the skin also known as "coke bugs". These symptoms can last for weeks or, in some cases, months. Even after most withdrawal symptoms dissipate most users feel the need to continue using the drug; this feeling can last for years and may peak during times of stress. About 30–40% of individuals with cocaine dependence will turn to other substances such as medication and alcohol after giving up cocaine. There are various medications on the market to ease cocaine withdrawal symptoms.

Risk

A study consisting of 1,081 U.S. residents who had first used cocaine within the previous 24 months was conducted. It was found that the risk of becoming dependent on cocaine within two years of first use was 5–6%. The risk of becoming dependent within 10 years of first use increased to 15–16%. These were the aggregate rates for all types of use considered, such as smoking, snorting, and injecting. Among recent-onset users individual rates of dependency were higher for smoking (3.4 times) and much higher for injecting. Women were 3.3 times more likely to become dependent, compared with men. Users who started at ages 12 or 13 were four times as likely to become dependent compared to those who started between ages 18 and 20.

However, a study of non-deviant users in Amsterdam found a "relative absence of destructive and compulsive use patterns over a ten year period" and concluded that cocaine users can and do exercise control. "Our respondents applied two basic types of controls to themselves: 1) restricting use to certain situations and to emotional states in which cocaine's effects would be most positive, and 2) limiting mode of ingestion to snorting of modest amounts of cocaine, staying below 2.5 grams a week for some, and below 0.5 grams a week for most. Nevertheless, those whose use level exceeded 2.5 grams a week all returned to lower levels."

Treatment

Therapy

Twelve-step programs such as Cocaine Anonymous (modeled on Alcoholics Anonymous) have been widely used to help those with cocaine addiction. Cognitive behavioral therapy (CBT) combined with motivational therapy (MT) have proven to be more helpful than 12 step programs in treating cocaine dependency. However, both these approaches have a fairly low success rate. Other non-pharmacological treatments such as acupuncture and hypnosis have been explored, but without conclusive results.

Medications

Numerous medications have been investigated for use in cocaine dependence, but as of 2015, none of them were considered to be effective. Anticonvulsants, such as carbamazepine, gabapentin, lamotrigine, and topiramate, do not appear to be effective as treatment. Limited evidence suggests that antipsychotics are also ineffective for treatment of cocaine dependence. Few studies have examined bupropion (a novel antidepressant) for cocaine dependence; however, trials performed thus far have not shown it to be an effective form of treatment for this purpose.

The National Institute on Drug Abuse (NIDA) of the U.S. National Institutes of Health is researching modafinil, a narcolepsy drug and mild stimulant, as a potential cocaine treatment. Ibogaine has been under investigation as a treatment for cocaine dependency and is used in clinics in Mexico, the Netherlands and Canada, but cannot be used legally in the United States. Other medications that have been investigated for this purpose include acetylcysteine, baclofen, and vanoxerine. Medications, such as phenelzine, have been used to cause an "aversion reaction" when administered with cocaine.

Nicotine

Nicotine is a potent parasympathomimetic stimulant and an alkaloid found in the nightshade family of plants. Nicotine acts as an agonist at most nicotinic acetylcholine receptors (nAChRs), except at two nicotinic receptor subunits (nAChRα9 and nAChRα10) where it acts as a receptor antagonist. Nicotine is found in the leaves of *Nicotiana rustica* in amounts of 2–14%, the tobacco plant *Nicotiana tabacum, Duboisia hopwoodii* and *Asclepias syriaca.*

Nicotine constitutes approximately 0.6–3.0% of the dry weight of tobacco. It also occurs in edible plants, especially Solanaceae such as eggplants, potatoes, and tomatoes, but at trace levels generally under 200 nanograms per gram, dry weight (less than .00002%). Nicotine functions as an antiherbivore chemical; consequently, nicotine was widely used as an insecticide in the past and neonicotinoids such as imidacloprid are currently widely used.

Nicotine is highly addictive. An average cigarette yields about 2 mg of absorbed nicotine, and in lesser doses of that order, the substance acts as a stimulant in mammals, while high amounts (50–100 mg) can be harmful. This stimulant effect is a contributing factor to the addictive properties of tobacco smoking. Nicotine's addictive nature includes psychoactive effects, drug-reinforced behavior, compulsive use, relapse after abstinence, physical dependence and tolerance.

Beyond addiction, both short and long-term nicotine exposure have not been established as dangerous to adults, except among certain vulnerable groups. At high-enough doses, nicotine is associated with poisonings and is potentially lethal. Nicotine as a tool for quitting smoking has a good safety history. There is inadequate research to show that nicotine itself is associated with cancer in humans. Nicotine in the form of nicotine replacement products is less of a cancer risk than smoking. Nicotine is linked to possible birth defects. During pregnancy, there are risks to the child later in life for type 2 diabetes, obesity, hypertension, neurobehavioral defects, respiratory dysfunction, and infertility. The use of electronic cigarettes, which are designed to be refilled with nicotine-containing e-liquid, has raised concerns over nicotine overdoses, especially with regard to the possibility of young children ingesting the liquids.

Psychoactive Effects

Nicotine's mood-altering effects are different by report: in particular it is both a stimulant and a relaxant. First causing a release of glucose from the liver and epinephrine (adrenaline) from the adrenal medulla, it causes stimulation. Users report feelings of relaxation, sharpness, calmness, and alertness. Like any stimulant, it may very rarely cause the often uncomfortable akathisia. By reducing the appetite and raising the metabolism, some smokers may lose weight as a consequence.

When a cigarette is smoked, nicotine-rich blood passes from the lungs to the brain within seven seconds and immediately stimulates nicotinic acetylcholine receptors; this indirectly promotes the release of many chemical messengers such as acetylcholine, norepinephrine, epinephrine, arginine vasopressin, serotonin, dopamine, and beta-endorphin in parts of the brain. Nicotine also extends the duration of positive effects of dopamine and increases the sensitivity of the brain's reward system to rewarding stimuli. Most cigarettes contain 1–3 milligrams of inhalable nicotine. Studies suggest that when smokers wish to achieve a stimulating effect, they take short quick puffs, which produce a low level of blood nicotine.

Nicotine is unusual in comparison to most drugs, as its profile changes from stimulant to sedative with increasing dosages, a phenomenon known as "Nesbitt's paradox" after the doctor who first described it in 1969. At very high doses it dampens neuronal activity.

Uses

Medical

The primary therapeutic use of nicotine is in treating nicotine dependence in order to eliminate smoking with the damage it does to health. Controlled levels of nicotine are given to patients through gums, dermal patches, lozenges, electronic/substitute cigarettes or nasal sprays in an effort to wean them off their dependence. Studies have found that these therapies increase the chance of success of quitting by 50 to 70%, though reductions in the population as a whole have not been demonstrated.

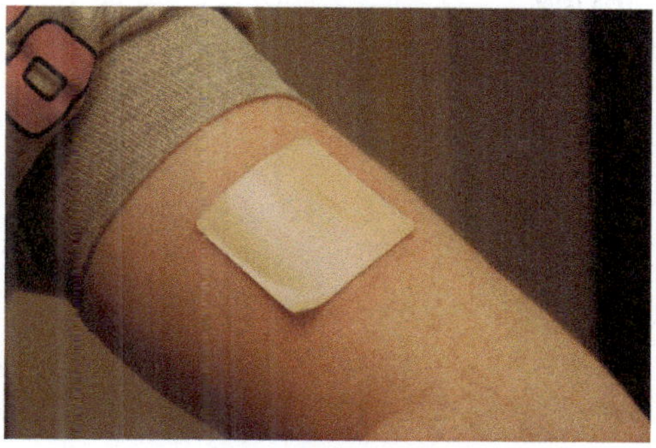

A 21 mg patch applied to the left arm. The Cochrane Collaboration finds that nicotine replacement therapy increases a quitter's chance of success by 50% to 70%.

Enhancing Performance

Nicotine is frequently used for its performance-enhancing effects on cognition, alertness, and focus. A meta-analysis of 41 double-blind, placebo-controlled studies concluded that nicotine or smoking had significant positive effects on aspects of fine motor abilities, alerting and orienting attention, and episodic and working memory. A 2015 review noted that stimulation of the α4β2 nicotinic receptor is responsible for certain improvements in attentional performance; among the nicotinic receptor subtypes, nicotine has the highest binding affinity at the α4β2 receptor (k_i=1 nM), which is also the biological target that mediates nicotine's addictive properties.

Recreational

Nicotine is commonly consumed as a recreational drug for its stimulant effects. Recreational nicotine products include chewing tobacco, cigars, cigarettes, e-cigarettes, snuff, pipe tobacco, and snus.

Adverse Effects

Limited data exists on the health effects of long-term use of pure nicotine, because nicotine is usually consumed via tobacco products. The long-term use of nicotine in the form of snus incurs a slight risk of cardiovascular disease compared to tobacco smoking and is not associated with cancer. Nicotine is one of the most rigorously studied drugs. The complex effects of nicotine are not entirely understood. Studies of continued use of nicotine replacement products in those who have stopped smoking found no adverse effects from months to several years, and that people with cardiovascular disease were able to tolerate them for 12 weeks. The general medical position is that nicotine itself poses few health risks, except among certain vulnerable groups. A 2016 Royal College of Physicians report found "nicotine alone in the doses used by smokers represents little if any hazard to the user". A 2014 American Heart Association policy statement found that some health concerns relate to nicotine. Experimental research suggests that adolescent nicotine use may harm brain development. Children exposed to nicotine may have a number of lifelong health issues. As medicine, nicotine is used to help with quitting smoking and has good safety in this form.

Vascular System

Human epidemiology studies show that nicotine use is not a significant cause of cardiovascular disease. A 2015 review found that nicotine is associated with cardiovascular disease. A 2016 review suggests that "the risks of nicotine without tobacco combustion products (cigarette smoke) are low compared to cigarette smoking, but are still of concern in people with cardiovascular disease." Some studies in people show the possibility that nicotine contributes to acute cardiovascular events in smokers with established cardiovascular disease, and induces pharmacologic effects that might contribute to increased atherosclerosis. Prolonged nicotine use seems not to increase atherosclerosis. Brief nicotine use, such as nicotine medicine, seems to incur a slight cardiovascular risk, even to people with established cardiovascular disease. A 2015 review found "Nicotine *in vitro* and in animal models can inhibit apoptosis and enhance angiogenesis, effects that raise concerns about the role of nicotine in promoting the acceleration of atherosclerotic disease." A 2012 Cochrane review found no evidence of an increased risk of cardiovascular disease with nicotine replacement products. A 1996 randomized controlled trial using nicotine patches found that serious adverse events were not more frequent among smokers with cardiovascular disease. A meta-analysis shows that snus consumption, which delivers nicotine at a dose equivalent to that of cigarettes, is not associated with heart attacks. Hence, it is not nicotine, but tobacco smoke's other components which seem to be implicated in ischemic heart disease. Nicotine increases heart rate and blood pressure and induces abnormal heart rhythms. Nicotine can also induce potentially atherogenic genes in human coronary artery endothelial cells. Microvascular injury can result through its action on nicotinic acetylcholine receptors (nAChRs). Nicotine does not adversely affect serum cholesterol levels, but a 2015 review found it may elevate serum cholesterol levels. Many quitting smoking studies using nicotine medicines report lowered dyslipidemia with considerable benefit in HDL/LDL ratios. Nicotine supports clot formation and aids in plaque formation by enhancing vascular smooth muscle.

Cancer

Although there is insufficient evidence to classify nicotine as a carcinogen, there is an ongoing debate about whether it functions as a tumor promoter. *In vitro* studies have associated it with cancer, but carcinogenicity has not been demonstrated *in vivo*. There is inadequate research to demonstrate that nicotine is associated with cancer in humans, but there is evidence indicating possible oral, esophageal, or pancreatic cancer risks. Nicotine in the form of nicotine replacement products is less of a cancer risk than smoking. Nicotine replacement products have not been shown to be associated with cancer in the real world.

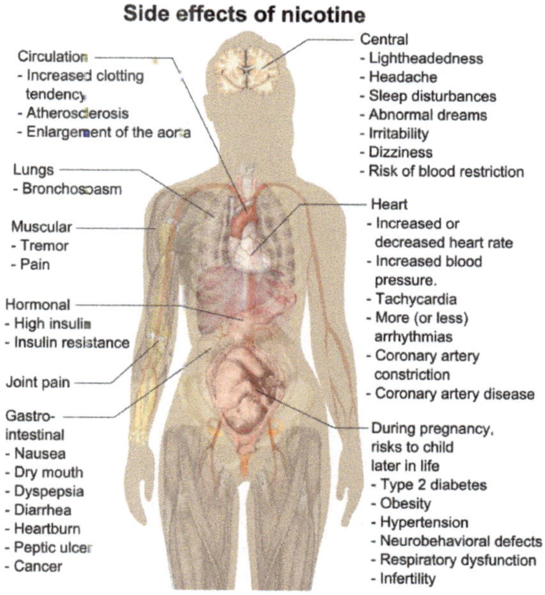

Possible side effects of nicotine.

While no epidemiological evidence directly supports the notion that nicotine acts as a carcinogen in the formation of human cancer, research has identified nicotine's indirect involvement in cancer formation in animal models and cell cultures. Nicotine increases cholinergic signalling and adrenergic signalling in the case of colon cancer, thereby impeding apoptosis (programmed cell death), promoting tumor growth, and activating growth factors and cellular mitogenic factors such as 5-lipoxygenase (5-LOX), and epidermal growth factor (EGF). Nicotine also promotes cancer growth by stimulating angiogenesis and neovascularization. In one study, nicotine administered to mice with tumors caused increases in tumor size (twofold increase), metastasis (nine-fold increase), and tumor recurrence (threefold increase). *N*-Nitrosonornicotine (NNN), classified by the International Agency for Research on Cancer (IARC) as a Group 1 carcinogen, has been shown to form *in vitro* from nornicotine in human saliva, indicating nornicotine is a carcinogen precursor. The IARC has not evaluated pure nicotine or assigned it to an official carcinogenic classification.

In cancer cells, nicotine promotes the epithelial–mesenchymal transition which makes the cancer cells more resistant to drugs that treat cancer.

Fetal Development

In pregnancy, a 2013 review noted that "nicotine is only 1 of more than 4000 compounds to which the fetus is exposed through maternal smoking. Of these, ~30 compounds have been associated with adverse health outcomes. Although the exact mechanisms by which nicotine produces adverse fetal effects are unknown, it is likely that hypoxia, undernourishment of the fetus, and direct vasoconstrictor effects on the placental and umbilical vessels all play a role. Nicotine also has been shown to have significant deleterious effects on brain development, including alterations in brain metabolism and neurotransmitter systems and abnormal brain development." It also notes that "abnormalities of newborn neurobehavior, including impaired orientation and autonomic regulation and abnormalities of muscle tone, have been identified in a number of prenatal nicotine exposure studies" and that there is weak data associating fetal nicotine exposure with newborn facial clefts, and that there is no good evidence for newborns suffering nicotine withdrawal from fetal exposure to nicotine.

Effective April 1, 1990, the Office of Environmental Health Hazard Assessment (OEHHA) of the California Environmental Protection Agency added nicotine to the list of chemicals known to cause developmental toxicity.

Nicotine is not safe to use in any amount during pregnancy . Questions exist regarding nicotine use during pregnancy and their potential consequences on fetal growth and mortality. Nicotine negatively affects pregnancy outcomes and fetal brain development. Risks to the child later in life via nicotine exposure during pregnancy include type 2 diabetes, obesity, hypertension, neurobehavioral defects, respiratory dysfunction, and infertility. Nicotine crosses the placenta and is found in the breast milk of mothers who smoke as well as mothers who inhale passive smoke.

Reinforcement Disorders

Nicotine dependence involves aspects of both psychological dependence and physical dependence, since discontinuation of extended use has been shown to produce both affective (e.g., anxiety, irritability, craving, anhedonia) and somatic (mild motor dysfunctions such as tremor) withdrawal symptoms. Withdrawal symptoms can persist for several weeks. Nicotine has clinically significant cognitive-enhancing effects at low doses, particularly in fine motor skills, attention, and memory. These beneficial cognitive effects may play a role in the maintenance of tobacco dependence.

Nicotine is highly addictive, comparable to heroin or cocaine. Nicotine activates the mesolimbic pathway and induces long-term ΔFosB expression in the nucleus accumbens when inhaled or injected at sufficiently high doses, but not necessarily when ingested. Consequently, repeated daily exposure (possibly excluding oral route) to nicotine can result in accumbal ΔFosB overexpression, in turn causing nicotine addiction.

In dependent smokers, smoking during withdrawal returns cognitive abilities to pre-withdrawal levels, but chronic use may not offer cognitive benefits over not smoking.

Connections to the Use of Other Substances

In animals it is relatively simple to determine if consumption of a certain drug increases the later attraction of another drug. In humans, where such direct experiments are not possible, longitudinal studies can show if the probability of a substance use is related to earlier use of other substances.

In mice nicotine increased the probability of later consumption of cocaine and the experiments permitted concrete conclusions on the underlying molecular biological alteration in the brain. The biological changes in mice correspond to the epidemiological observations in humans that nicotine consumption is coupled to an increased probability of later use of cannabis and cocaine.

In rats cannabis consumption – earlier in life – increased the later self-administration of nicotine. A study of drug use of 14,577 US 12th graders showed that alcohol consumption was associated with an increased probability of later use of tobacco, cannabis, and other illegal drugs.

Overdose

Nicotine is regarded as a potentially lethal poison. The LD_{50} of nicotine is 50 mg/kg for rats and 3 mg/kg for mice. 30–60 mg (0.5–1.0 mg/kg) can be a lethal dosage for adult humans. However, the widely used human LD_{50} estimate of 0.5–1.0 mg/kg was questioned in a 2013 review, in light of several documented cases of humans surviving much higher doses; the 2013 review suggests that the lower limit causing fatal outcomes is 500–1000 mg of ingested nicotine, corresponding to 6.5–13 mg/kg orally. Nevertheless, nicotine has a relatively high toxicity in comparison to many other alkaloids such as caffeine, which has an LD_{50} of 127 mg/kg when administered to mice.

At high-enough doses, it is associated with nicotine poisoning. Today nicotine is less commonly used in agricultural insecticides, which was a main source of poisoning. More recent cases of poisoning typically appear to be in the form of Green Tobacco Sickness or due to accidental ingestion of tobacco or tobacco products or ingestion of nicotine containing plants. People who harvest or cultivate tobacco may experience Green Tobacco Sickness (GTS), a type of nicotine poisoning caused by dermal exposure to wet tobacco leaves. This occurs most commonly in young, inexperienced tobacco harvesters who do not consume tobacco. People can be exposed to nicotine in the workplace by breathing it in, skin absorption, swallowing it, or eye contact. The Occupational Safety and Health Administration (OSHA) has set the legal limit (permissible exposure limit) for nicotine exposure in the workplace as 0.5 mg/m^3 skin exposure over an 8-hour workday. The US National Institute for Occupational Safety and Health (NIOSH) has set a recommended exposure limit (REL) of 0.5 mg/m^3 skin exposure over an 8-hour workday. At environmental levels of 5 mg/m^3, nicotine is immediately dangerous to life and health.

It is unlikely that a person would overdose on nicotine through smoking alone. The US Food and Drug Administration (FDA) stated in 2013 that "There are no significant safety concerns associated with using more than one OTC NRT at the same time, or using an OTC NRT at the same time as another nicotine-containing product—including a cigarette."

The recent rise in the use of electronic cigarettes, many forms of which are designed to be refilled with nicotine-containing e-liquid supplied in small plastic bottles, has raised concerns over nicotine overdoses, especially in the possibility of young children ingesting the liquids. A 2015 Public Health England report noted an "unconfirmed newspaper report of a fatal poisoning of a two-year old child" and two published case reports of children of similar age who had recovered after ingesting e-liquid and vomiting. They also noted case reports of suicides by nicotine. Where adults drank liquid containing up to 1,500 mg of nicotine they recovered (helped by vomiting), but an ingestion apparently of about 10,000 mg was fatal, as was an injection. They commented that "Serious nicotine poisoning seems normally prevented by the fact that relatively low doses of nicotine cause nausea and vomiting, which stops users from further intake."

Pharmacology

Pharmacodynamics

Nicotine acts as a receptor agonist at most nicotinic acetylcholine receptors (nAChRs), except at two nicotinic receptor subunits (nAChRα9 and nAChRα10) where it acts as a receptor antagonist.

Central Nervous System

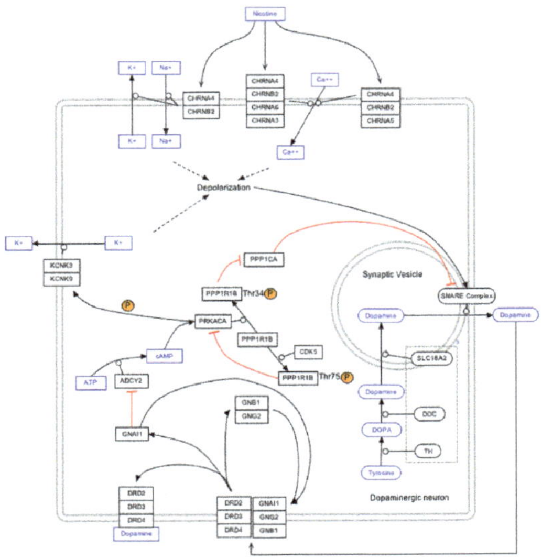

Effect of nicotine on dopaminergic neurons.

By binding to nicotinic acetylcholine receptors in the brain, nicotine elicits its psychoactive effects and increases the levels of several neurotransmitters in various brain structures – acting as a sort of "volume control." Nicotine has a higher affinity for nicotinic receptors in the brain than those in skeletal muscle, though at toxic doses it can induce contractions and respiratory paralysis. Nicotine's selectivity is thought to be due to a particular amino acid difference on these receptor subtypes.

Nicotine activates nicotinic receptors (particularly α4β2 nicotinic receptors) on neurons that innervate the ventral tegmental area and within the mesolimbic pathway where it appears to cause the release of dopamine. This nicotine-induced dopamine release occurs at least partially through activation of the cholinergic–dopaminergic reward link in the ventral tegmental area. Nicotine also appears to induce the release of endogenous opioids that activate opioid pathways in the reward system, since naltrexone – an opioid receptor antagonist – blocks nicotine self-administration. These actions are largely responsible for the strongly reinforcing effects of nicotine, which often occur in the absence of euphoria; however, mild euphoria from nicotine use can occur in some individuals. Chronic nicotine use inhibits class I and II histone deacetylases in the striatum, where this effect plays a role in nicotine addiction.

Sympathetic Nervous System

Nicotine also activates the sympathetic nervous system, acting via splanchnic nerves to the adrenal medulla, stimulating the release of epinephrine. Acetylcholine released by preganglionic sympathetic fibers of these nerves acts on nicotinic acetylcholine receptors, causing the release of epinephrine (and norepinephrine) into the bloodstream. Nicotine also has an affinity for melanin-containing tissues due to its precursor function in melanin synthesis or due to the irreversible binding of melanin and nicotine. This has been suggested to underlie the increased nicotine dependence and lower smoking cessation rates in darker pigmented individuals. However, further research is warranted before a definite conclusive link can be inferred.

Adrenal Medulla

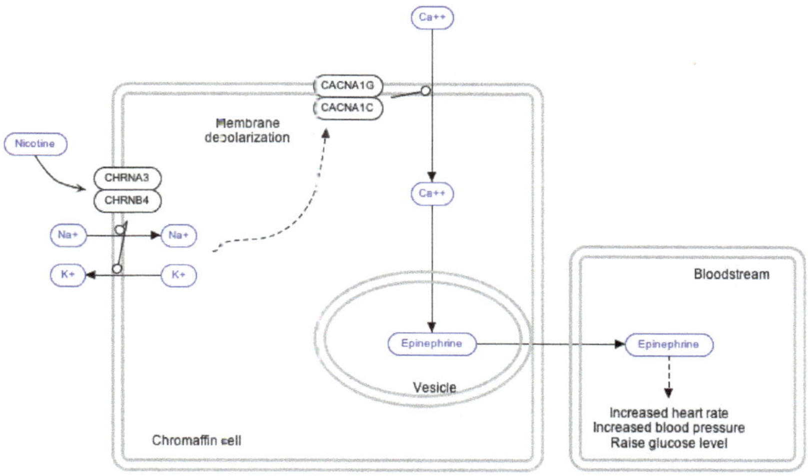

Effect of nicotine on chromaffin cells.

By binding to ganglion type nicotinic receptors in the adrenal medulla, nicotine increases flow of adrenaline (epinephrine), a stimulating hormone and neurotransmitter. By binding to the receptors, it causes cell depolarization and an influx of calcium through voltage-gated calcium channels. Calcium triggers the exocytosis of chromaffin granules and thus the release of epinephrine (and norepinephrine) into the bloodstream. The release of epinephrine (adrenaline) causes an increase in heart rate, blood pressure and respiration, as well as higher blood glucose levels.

Nicotine has a half-life of 1–2 hours. Cotinine is an active metabolite of nicotine that remains in the blood with a half-life of 18–20 hours, making it easier to analyze.

Pharmacokinetics

As nicotine enters the body, it is distributed quickly through the bloodstream and crosses the blood–brain barrier reaching the brain within 10–20 seconds after inhalation. The elimination half-life of nicotine in the body is around two hours.

The amount of nicotine absorbed by the body from smoking can depend on many factors, including the types of tobacco, whether the smoke is inhaled, and whether a filter is used. However, it has been found that the nicotine yield of individual products has only a small effect (4.4%) on the blood concentration of nicotine, suggesting "the assumed health advantage of switching to lower-tar and lower-nicotine cigarettes may be largely offset by the tendency of smokers to compensate by increasing inhalation".

Nicotine is metabolized in the liver by cytochrome P450 enzymes (mostly CYP2A6, and also by CYP2B6) and FMO3, which selectively metabolizes (*S*)-nicotine. A major metabolite is cotinine. Other primary metabolites include nicotine *N'*-oxide, nornicotine, nicotine isomethonium ion, 2-hydroxynicotine and nicotine glucuronide. Under some conditions, other substances may be formed such as myosmine.

Glucuronidation and oxidative metabolism of nicotine to cotinine are both inhibited by menthol, an additive to mentholated cigarettes, thus increasing the half-life of nicotine *in vivo*.

Chemistry

Nicotine is a hygroscopic, colorless to yellow-brown, oily liquid, that is readily soluble in alcohol, ether or light petroleum. It is miscible with water in its base form between 60 °C and 210 °C. As a nitrogenous base, nicotine forms salts with acids that are usually solid and water-soluble. Its flash point is 95 °C and its auto-ignition temperature is 244 °C.

Nicotine is readily volatile (vapor pressure 5.5 Pa at 25 ℃) and dibasic ($K_{b1} = 1\times10^{-6}$, $K_{b2} = 1\times10^{-11}$).

Nicotine is optically active, having two enantiomeric forms. The naturally occurring form of nicotine is levorotatory with a specific rotation of $[\alpha]_D = -166.4°$ ((−)-nicotine).

The dextrorotatory form, (+)-nicotine is physiologically less active than (–)-nicotine. (–)-nicotine is more toxic than (+)-nicotine. The salts of (+)-nicotine are usually dextrorotatory. The hydrochloride and sulphate salts become optically inactive if heated in a closed vessel above 180 °C.

On exposure to ultraviolet light or various oxidizing agents, nicotine is converted to nicotine oxide, nicotinic acid (vitamin B3), and methylamine.

Occurrence and Biosynthesis

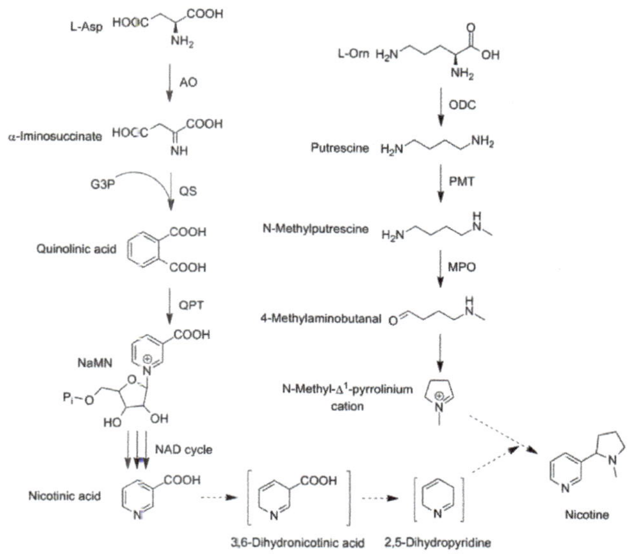

Nicotine biosynthesis

Nicotine is a natural product of tobacco, occurring in the leaves in a range of 0.5 to 7.5% depending on variety. Nicotine also naturally occurs in smaller amounts in plants from the family Solanaceae (such as potatoes, tomatoes, and eggplant).

The biosynthetic pathway of nicotine involves a coupling reaction between the two cyclic structures that compose nicotine. Metabolic studies show that the pyridine ring of nicotine is derived from niacin (nicotinic acid) while the pyrrolidone is derived from *N*-methyl-Δ^1-pyrrollidium cation. Biosynthesis of the two component structures proceeds via two independent syntheses, the NAD pathway for niacin and the tropane pathway for *N*-methyl-Δ^1-pyrrollidium cation.

The NAD pathway in the genus *nicotiana* begins with the oxidation of aspartic acid into α-imino succinate by aspartate oxidase (AO). This is followed by a condensation with glyceraldehyde-3-phosphate and a cyclization catalyzed by quinolinate synthase (QS) to give quinolinic acid. Quinolinic acid then reacts with phosphoriboxyl pyrophosphate catalyzed by quinolinic acid phosphoribosyl transferase (QPT) to form niacin mononucleotide (NaMN). The reaction now proceeds via the NAD salvage cycle to produce niacin via the conversion of nicotinamide by the enzyme nicotinamidase.

The *N*-methyl-Δ^1-pyrrollidium cation used in the synthesis of nicotine is an intermediate in the synthesis of tropane-derived alkaloids. Biosynthesis begins with decarboxylation of ornithine by ornithine decarboxylase (ODC) to produce putrescine. Putrescine is then converted into *N*-methyl putrescine via methylation by SAM catalyzed by putrescine *N*-methyltransferase (PMT). *N*-methylputrescine then undergoes deamination into 4-methylaminobutanal by the *N*-methylputrescine oxidase (MPO) enzyme, 4-methylaminobutanal then spontaneously cyclize into *N*-methyl-Δ^1-pyrrollidium cation.

The final step in the synthesis of nicotine is the coupling between *N*-methyl-Δ^1-pyrrollidium cation and niacin. Although studies conclude some form of coupling between the two component structures, the definite process and mechanism remains undetermined. The current agreed theory involves the conversion of niacin into 2,5-dihydropyridine through 3,6-dihydronicotinic acid. The 2,5-dihydropyridine intermediate would then react with *N*-methyl-Δ^1-pyrrollidium cation to form enantiomerically pure (−)-nicotine.

Detection in Body Fluids

Nicotine can be quantified in blood, plasma, or urine to confirm a diagnosis of poisoning or to facilitate a medicolegal death investigation. Urinary or salivary cotinine concentrations are frequently measured for the purposes of pre-employment and health insurance medical screening programs. Careful interpretation of results is important, since passive exposure to cigarette smoke can result in significant accumulation of nicotine, followed by the appearance of its metabolites in various body fluids. Nicotine use is not regulated in competitive sports programs.

History

Nicotine is named after the tobacco plant *Nicotiana tabacum,* which in turn is named after the French ambassador in Portugal, Jean Nicot de Villemain, who sent tobacco and seeds to Paris in 1560, presented to the French King, and who promoted their medicinal use. Smoking was believed to protect against illness, particularly the plague.

Tobacco was introduced to Europe in 1559, and by the late 17th century, it was used not only for smoking but also as an insecticide. After World War II, over 2,500 tons of nicotine insecticide were used worldwide, but by the 1980s the use of nicotine insecticide had declined below 200 tons. This was due to the availability of other insecticides that are cheaper and less harmful to mammals.

Currently, nicotine, even in the form of tobacco dust, is prohibited as a pesticide for organic farming in the United States.

In 2008, the EPA received a request, from the registrant, to cancel the registration of the last nicotine pesticide registered in the United States. This request was granted, and since 1 January 2014, this pesticide has not been available for sale.

Chemical Identification

Nicotine was first isolated from the tobacco plant in 1828 by physician Wilhelm Heinrich Posselt and chemist Karl Ludwig Reimann of Germany, who considered it a poison. Its chemical empirical formula was described by Melsens in 1843, its structure was discovered by Adolf Pinner and Richard Wolffenstein in 1893, and it was first synthesized by Amé Pictet and A. Rotschy in 1904.

Society and Culture

The nicotine content of popular American-brand cigarettes has slowly increased over the years, and one study found that there was an average increase of 1.78% per year between the years of 1998 and 2005.

Research

While acute/initial nicotine intake causes activation of nicotine receptors, chronic low doses of nicotine use leads to desensitisation of nicotine receptors (due to the development of tolerance) and results in an antidepressant effect, with research showing low dose nicotine patches being an effective treatment of major depressive disorder in non-smokers. However, the original research concluded that: "Nicotine patches produced short-term improvement of depression with minor side effects. Because of nicotine's high risk to health, nicotine patches are not recommended for clinical use in depression."

Though tobacco smoking is associated with an increased risk of Alzheimer's disease, there is evidence that nicotine itself has the potential to prevent and treat Alzheimer's disease.

Research into nicotine's most predominant metabolite, cotinine, suggests that some of nicotine's psychoactive effects are mediated by cotinine.

Little research is available in humans but animal research suggests there is potential benefit from nicotine in Parkinson's disease.

There is tentative evidence that nicotinamides may improve depression.

Alcoholism

Alcoholism, also known as alcohol use disorder (AUD), is a broad term for any drinking of alcohol that results in mental or physical health problems. It was previously divided into two types: alcohol abuse and alcohol dependence. In a medical context, alcoholism is said to exist when two or more of the following conditions is present:

a person drinks large amounts over a long time period, has difficulty cutting down, acquiring and drinking alcohol takes up a great deal of time, alcohol is strongly desired, usage results in not fulfilling responsibilities, usage results in social problems, usage results in health problems, usage results in risky situations, withdrawal occurs when stopping, and alcohol tolerance has occurred with use. Risky situations include drinking and driving or having unsafe sex among others. Alcohol use can affect all parts of the body but particularly affects the brain, heart, liver, pancreas, and immune system. This can result in mental illness, Wernicke–Korsakoff syndrome, an irregular heart beat, liver failure, and an increase in the risk of cancer, among other diseases. Drinking during pregnancy can cause damage to the baby resulting in fetal alcohol spectrum disorders. Generally women are more sensitive to alcohol's harmful physical and mental effects than men.

Both environmental factors and genetics are associated with alcoholism with about half the risk attributed to each. A person with a parent or sibling with alcoholism is three to four times more likely to be alcoholic themselves. Environmental factors include social, cultural, and behavioral influences. High stress levels, anxiety, as well as inexpensive easily accessible alcohol increases risk. People may continue to drink partly to prevent or improve symptoms of withdrawal. A low level of withdrawal may last for months following stopping. Medically, alcoholism is considered both a physical and mental illness. Both questionnaires and certain blood tests may detect people with possible alcoholism. Further information is then collected to confirm the diagnosis.

Prevention of alcoholism may be attempted by regulating and limiting the sale of alcohol, taxing alcohol to increase its cost, and providing inexpensive treatment. Treatment may take several steps. Because of the medical problems that can occur during withdrawal, alcohol detoxification should be carefully controlled. One common method involves the use of benzodiazepine medications, such as diazepam. This can be either given while admitted to a health care institution or occasionally while a person remains in the community with close supervision. Other addictions or mental illness may complicate treatment. After detoxification support such as group therapy or support groups are used to help keep a person from returning to drinking. One commonly used form of support is the group Alcoholics Anonymous. The medications acamprosate, disulfiram, or naltrexone may also be used to help prevent further drinking.

The World Health Organization estimates that as of 2010 there were 208 million people with alcoholism worldwide (4.1% of the population over 15 years of age). In the United States about 17 million (7%) of adults and 0.7 million (2.8%) of those age 12 to 17 years of age are affected. It is more common among males and young adults, becoming less common in middle and old age. It is the least common in Africa at 1.1% and has the highest rates in Eastern Europe at 11%. Alcoholism directly resulted in 139,000 deaths in 2013 up from 112,000 deaths in 1990. A total of 3.3 million deaths (5.9% of all deaths) are believed to be due to alcohol. It often reduces a person's life expectancy by around ten years. In the United States it resulted in economic costs of $224 billion USD in 2006. Many terms, some insulting and others informal, have been used to refer to people affected by alcoholism including: tippler, drunkard, dipsomaniac, and souse. In 1979, the World Health Organization discouraged the use of "alcoholism" due to its inexact meaning, preferring "alcohol dependence syndrome".

Early Signs

The risk of alcohol dependence begins at low levels of drinking and increases directly with both the volume of alcohol consumed and a pattern of drinking larger amounts on an occasion, to the point of intoxication, which is sometimes called "binge drinking". Young adults are particularly at risk of engaging in binge drinking.

Long-term Misuse

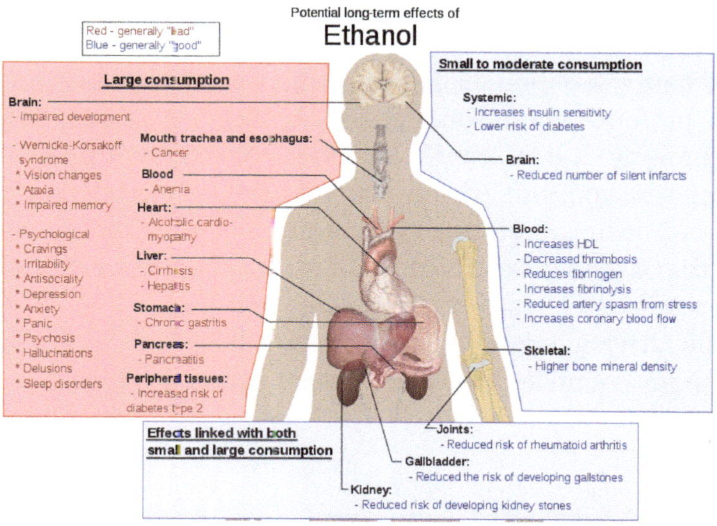

Some of the possible long-term effects of ethanol an individual may develop. Additionally, in pregnant women, alcohol can cause fetal alcohol syndrome.

Alcoholism is characterised by an increased tolerance to alcohol–which means that an individual can consume more alcohol–and physical dependence on alcohol, which makes it hard for an individual to control their consumption. The physical dependency caused by alcohol can lead to an affected individual having a very strong urge to drink alcohol. These characteristics play a role decreasing an alcoholic's ability to stop drinking. Alcoholism can have adverse effects on mental health, causing psychiatric disorders and increasing the risk of suicide. A depressed mood is a common symptom of heavy alcohol drinkers.

Warning Signs

Warning signs of alcoholism include the consumption of increasing amounts of alcohol and frequent intoxication, preoccupation with drinking to the exclusion of other activities, promises to quit drinking and failure to keep them, the inability to remember what was said or done while drinking (colloquially known as "blackouts"), personality changes associated with drinking, denial or the making of excuses for drinking, the refusal to admit excessive drinking, dysfunction or other problems at work or school, the loss of interest in personal appearance or hygiene, marital and economic problems, and the complaint of poor health, with loss of appetite, respiratory infections, or increased anxiety.

Physical

Short-term Effects

Drinking enough to cause a blood alcohol concentration (BAC) of 0.03–0.12% typically causes an overall improvement in mood and possible euphoria (a "happy" feeling), increased self-confidence and sociability, decreased anxiety, a flushed, red appearance in the face and impaired judgment and fine muscle coordination. A BAC of 0.09% to 0.25% causes lethargy, sedation, balance problems and blurred vision. A BAC of 0.18% to 0.30% causes profound confusion, impaired speech (e.g. slurred speech), staggering, dizziness and vomiting. A BAC from 0.25% to 0.40% causes stupor, unconsciousness, anterograde amnesia, vomiting (death may occur due to inhalation of vomit (pulmonary aspiration) while unconscious and respiratory depression (potentially life-threatening). A BAC from 0.35% to 0.80% causes a coma (unconsciousness), life-threatening respiratory depression and possibly fatal alcohol poisoning. With all alcoholic beverages, drinking while driving, operating an aircraft or heavy machinery increases the risk of an accident; many countries have penalties for drunk driving.

Long-term Effects

Drinking more than one drink a day for women or two drinks for men increases the risk of heart disease, high blood pressure, atrial fibrillation, and stroke. Risk is greater in younger people due to binge drinking which may result in violence or accidents. About 3.3 million deaths (5.9% of all deaths) are believed to be due to alcohol each year. Alcoholism reduces a person's life expectancy by around ten years and alcohol use is the third leading cause of early death in the United States. No professional medical association recommends that people who are nondrinkers should start drinking wine. Long-term alcohol abuse can cause a number of physical symptoms, including cirrhosis of the liver, pancreatitis, epilepsy, polyneuropathy, alcoholic dementia, heart disease, nutritional deficiencies, peptic ulcers and sexual dysfunction, and can eventually be fatal. Other physical effects include an increased risk of developing cardiovascular disease, malabsorption, alcoholic liver disease, and cancer. Damage to the central nervous system and peripheral nervous system can occur from sustained alcohol consumption. A wide range of immunologic defects can result and there may be a generalized skeletal fragility, in addition to a recognized tendency to accidental injury, resulting a propensity to bone fractures.

Women develop long-term complications of alcohol dependence more rapidly than do men. Additionally, women have a higher mortality rate from alcoholism than men. Examples of long-term complications include brain, heart, and liver damage and an increased risk of breast cancer. Additionally, heavy drinking over time has been found to have a negative effect on reproductive functioning in women. This results in reproductive dysfunction such as anovulation, decreased ovarian mass, problems or irregularity of the menstrual cycle, and early menopause. Alcoholic ketoacidosis can occur in individuals who chronically abuse alcohol and have a recent history of binge drinking. The amount of alcohol that can be biologically processed and its effects differ between sexes. Equal dosages of alcohol consumed by men and women generally result in women having higher blood alcohol concentrations (BACs), since women generally have a higher percentage of body fat and therefore a lower volume of distribution for alcohol than men, and because the stomachs of men tend to metabolize alcohol more quickly.

Psychiatric

Long-term misuse of alcohol can cause a wide range of mental health problems. Severe cognitive problems are common; approximately 10 percent of all dementia cases are related to alcohol consumption, making it the second leading cause of dementia. Excessive alcohol use causes damage to brain function, and psychological health can be increasingly affected over time. Social skills are significantly impaired in people suffering from alcoholism due to the neurotoxic effects of alcohol on the brain, especially the prefrontal cortex area of the brain. The social skills that are impaired by alcohol abuse include impairments in perceiving facial emotions, prosody perception problems and theory of mind deficits; the ability to understand humour is also impaired in alcohol abusers. Psychiatric disorders are common in alcoholics, with as many as 25 percent suffering severe psychiatric disturbances. The most prevalent psychiatric symptoms are anxiety and depression disorders. Psychiatric symptoms usually initially worsen during alcohol withdrawal, but typically improve or disappear with continued abstinence. Psychosis, confusion, and organic brain syndrome may be caused by alcohol misuse, which can lead to a misdiagnosis such as schizophrenia. Panic disorder can develop or worsen as a direct result of long-term alcohol misuse.

The co-occurrence of major depressive disorder and alcoholism is well documented. Among those with comorbid occurrences, a distinction is commonly made between depressive episodes that remit with alcohol abstinence ("substance-induced"), and depressive episodes that are primary and do not remit with abstinence ("independent" episodes). Additional use of other drugs may increase the risk of depression. Psychiatric disorders differ depending on gender. Women who have alcohol-use disorders often have a co-occurring psychiatric diagnosis such as major depression, anxiety, panic disorder, bulimia, post-traumatic stress disorder (PTSD), or borderline personality disorder. Men with alcohol-use disorders more often have a co-occurring diagnosis of narcissistic or antisocial personality disorder, bipolar disorder, schizophrenia, impulse disorders or attention deficit/hyperactivity disorder (ADHD). Women with alcoholism are more likely to experience physical or sexual assault, abuse and domestic violence than women in the general population, which can lead to higher instances of psychiatric disorders and greater dependence on alcohol.

Social Effects

The social problems arising from alcoholism are serious, caused by the pathological changes in the brain and the intoxicating effects of alcohol. Alcohol abuse is associated with an increased risk of committing criminal offences, including child abuse, domestic violence, rape, burglary and assault. Alcoholism is associated with loss of employment, which can lead to financial problems. Drinking at inappropriate times, and behavior caused by reduced judgment, can lead to legal consequences, such as criminal charges for drunk driving or public disorder, or civil penalties for tortious behavior, and may lead to a criminal sentence. An alcoholic's behavior and mental impairment, while drunk, can profoundly affect those surrounding them and lead to isolation from family and friends. This isolation can lead to marital conflict and divorce, or contribute to domestic violence. Alcoholism can also lead to child neglect, with subsequent lasting damage to the emotional development of the alcoholic's children. For this reason, children of alcoholic parents can develop a number of emotional problems. For example, they can become afraid of their parents, because of their unstable mood behaviors. In addition, they can develop considerable amount of shame over their inadequacy to liberate their parents from alcoholism. As a result of this failure, they develop wretched self-images, which can lead to depression.

Alcohol Withdrawal

As with similar substances with a sedative-hypnotic mechanism, such as barbiturates and benzodiazepines, withdrawal from alcohol dependence can be fatal if it is not properly managed. Alcohol's primary effect is the increase in stimulation of the $GABA_A$ receptor, promoting central nervous system depression. With repeated heavy consumption of alcohol, these receptors are desensitized and reduced in number, resulting in tolerance and physical dependence. When alcohol consumption is stopped too abruptly, the person's nervous system suffers from uncontrolled synapse firing. This can result in symptoms that include anxiety, life-threatening seizures, delirium tremens, hallucinations, shakes and possible heart failure. Other neurotransmitter systems are also involved, especially dopamine, NMDA and glutamate.

Severe acute withdrawal symptoms such as delirium tremens and seizures rarely occur after 1-week post cessation of alcohol. The acute withdrawal phase can be defined as lasting between one and three weeks. In the period of 3–6 weeks following cessation increased anxiety, depression, as well as sleep disturbance, is common; fatigue and tension can persist for up to 5 weeks as part of the post-acute withdrawal syndrome; about a quarter of alcoholics experience anxiety and depression for up to 2 years. These post-acute withdrawal symptoms have also been demonstrated in animal models of alcohol dependence and withdrawal. A kindling effect also occurs in alcoholics whereby each subsequent withdrawal syndrome is more severe than the previous withdrawal episode; this is due to neuroadaptations which occur as a result of periods of abstinence followed by re-exposure to alcohol. Individuals who have had multiple withdrawal episodes are more likely to develop seizures and experience more severe anxiety during withdrawal from alcohol than alcohol-dependent individuals without a history of past alcohol withdrawal episodes. The kindling effect leads to persistent functional changes in brain neural circuits as well as to gene expression. Kindling also results in the intensification of psychological symptoms of alcohol withdrawal. There are decision tools and questionnaires which help guide physicians in evaluating alcohol withdrawal. For example, the CIWA-Ar objectifies alcohol withdrawal symptoms in order to guide therapy decisions which allows for an efficient interview while at the same time retaining clinical usefulness, validity, and reliability, ensuring proper care for withdrawal patients, who can be in danger of death.

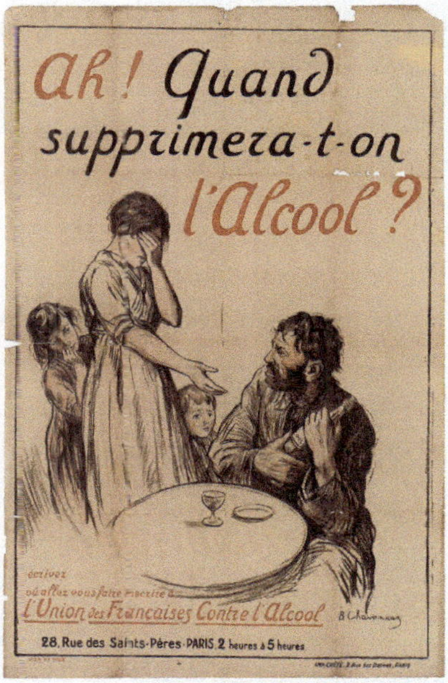

A French temperance poster from the Union des Françaises contre l'Alcool (this translates as "Union of French People Against Alcohol"). The poster states "Ah! Quand supprimera-t'on l'alcool?", which translates as "Ah! When will we [the nation] abolish alcohol?"

Causes

A complex mixture of genetic and environmental factors influences the risk of the development of alcoholism. Genes that influence the metabolism of alcohol also influence the risk of alcoholism, and may be indicated by a family history of alcoholism. One paper has found that alcohol use at an early age may influence the expression of genes which increase the risk of alcohol dependence. Individuals who have a genetic disposition to alcoholism are also more likely to begin drinking at an earlier age than average. Also, a younger age of onset of drinking is associated with an increased risk of the development of alcoholism, and about 40 percent of alcoholics will drink excessively by their late adolescence. It is not entirely clear whether this association is causal, and some researchers have been known to disagree with this view.

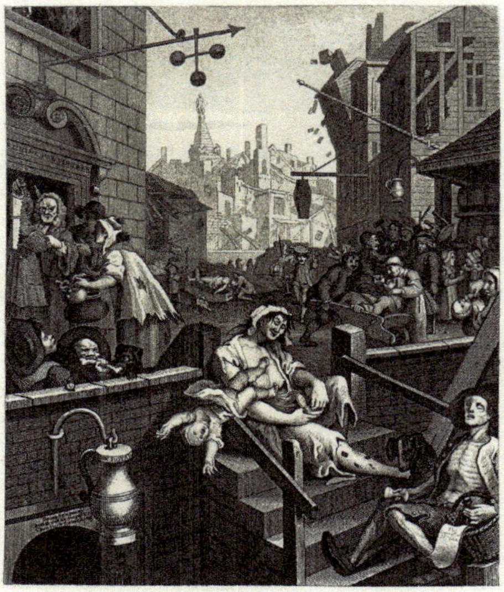

William Hogarth's *Gin Lane*, 1751

Severe childhood trauma is also associated with a general increase in the risk of drug dependency. Lack of peer and family support is associated with an increased risk of alcoholism developing. Genetics and adolescence are associated with an increased sensitivity to the neurotoxic effects of chronic alcohol abuse. Cortical degeneration due to the neurotoxic effects increases impulsive behaviour, which may contribute to the development, persistence and severity of alcohol use disorders. There is evidence that with abstinence, there is a reversal of at least some of the alcohol induced central nervous system damage. The use of cannabis was associated with later problems with alcohol use. Alcohol use was associated with an increased probability of later use of tobacco, cannabis, and other illegal drugs.

Availability

Alcohol is the most available, widely consumed, and widely abused recreational drug. Beer alone is the world's most widely consumed alcoholic beverage; it is the third-most popular drink overall, after water and tea. It is thought by some to be the oldest fermented beverage.

Gender Difference

Based on combined data from SAMHSA's 2004–2005 National Surveys on Drug Use & Health, the rate of past-year alcohol dependence or abuse among persons aged 12 or older varied by level of alcohol use: 44.7% of past month heavy drinkers, 18.5%

binge drinkers, 3.8% past month non-binge drinkers, and 1.3% of those who did not drink alcohol in the past month met the criteria for alcohol dependence or abuse in the past year. Males had higher rates than females for all measures of drinking in the past month: any alcohol use (57.5% vs. 45%), binge drinking (30.8% vs. 15.1%), and heavy alcohol use (10.5% vs. 3.3%), and males were twice as likely as females to have met the criteria for alcohol dependence or abuse in the past year (10.5% vs. 5.1%).

Genetic Variation

Genetic differences exist between different racial groups which affect the risk of developing alcohol dependence. For example, there are differences between African, East Asian and Indo-racial groups in how they metabolize alcohol. These genetic factors are believed to, in part, explain the differing rates of alcohol dependence among racial groups. The alcohol dehydrogenase allele ADH1 B*3 causes a more rapid metabolism of alcohol. The allele ADH1 B*3 is only found in those of African descent and certain Native American tribes. African Americans and Native Americans with this allele have a reduced risk of developing alcoholism. Native Americans however, have a significantly higher rate of alcoholism than average; it is unclear why this is the case. Other risk factors such as cultural environmental effects e.g. trauma have been proposed to explain the higher rates of alcoholism among Native Americans compared to alcoholism levels in caucasians.

A genome-wide association study of more than 100,000 human individuals identified variants of the gene *KLB*, which encodes the transmembrane protein β-Klotho, as highly associated with alcohol consumption. The protein β-Klotho is an essential element in cell surface receptors for hormones involved in modulation of appetites for simple sugars and alcohol.

Diagnosis

Definition

Misuse, problem use, abuse, and heavy use of alcohol refer to improper use of alcohol which may cause physical, social, or moral harm to the drinker. Moderate use is defined by *The Dietary Guidelines for Americans* as no more than two alcoholic beverages a day for men and no more than one alcoholic beverage a day for women. Some drinkers may drink more than 600 ml of alcohol per day during a heavy drinking period. The National Institute on Alcohol Abuse and Alcoholism (NIAAA) defines binge drinking as the amount of alcohol leading to a blood alcohol content (BAC) of 0.08, which, for most adults, would be reached by consuming five drinks for men or four for women over a two-hour period. According to the NIAAA, men may be at risk for alcohol-related problems if their alcohol consumption exceeds 14 standard drinks per week or 4 drinks per day, and women may be at risk if they have more than 7 standard drinks per week or 3 drinks per day. It defines a standard drink as one 12-ounce bottle of beer, one 5-ounce glass of wine, or 1.5 ounces of distilled spirits. Despite this risk, a 2014 report in the National Survey on

Drug Use and Health found that only 10% of either "heavy drinkers" or "binge drinkers" defined according to the above criteria also met the criteria for alcohol dependence, while only 1.3% of non-binge drinkers met the criteria. An inference drawn from this study is that evidence-based policy strategies and clinical preventive services may effectively reduce binge drinking without requiring addiction treatment in most cases.

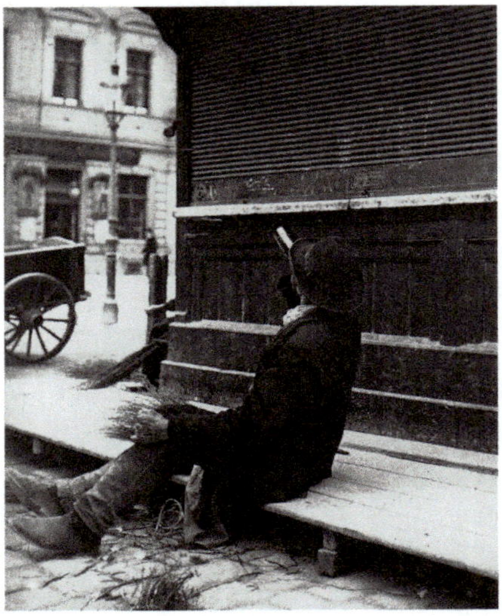

A picture of a man drinking from a bottle of alcohol while sitting on a boardwalk, ca. 1905–1914. Picture by Austrian photographer Emil Mayer.

Alcoholism

The term *alcoholism* is commonly used amongst laypeople, but it is poorly defined. The WHO calls *alcoholism* "a term of long-standing use and variable meaning", and use of the term was disfavored by a 1979 WHO expert committee. *The Big Book* (from Alcoholics Anonymous) states that once a person is an alcoholic, they are always an alcoholic, but does not define what is meant by the term *alcoholic* in this context. In 1960, Bill W., co-founder of Alcoholics Anonymous (AA), said:

> We have never called alcoholism a disease because, technically speaking, it is not a disease entity. For example, there is no such thing as heart disease. Instead there are many separate heart ailments, or combinations of them. It is something like that with alcoholism. Therefore we did not wish to get in wrong with the medical profession by pronouncing alcoholism a disease entity. Therefore we always called it an illness, or a malady—a far safer term for us to use. In professional and research contexts, the term "alcoholism" sometimes encompasses both alcohol abuse and alcohol dependence, and sometimes is considered equivalent to alcohol dependence. Talbot (1989) observes that alcoholism in the classical disease model follows a progressive course: if a person continues to drink, their condition will worsen. This will lead to harmful consequences in their life, physically, mentally, emotionally and socially.

Johnson'S Typologies

Johnson (1980) explores the emotional progression of the addict's response to alcohol. He looks at this in four phases. The first two are considered "normal" drinking and the last two are viewed as "typical" alcoholic drinking. Johnson's four phases consist of:

1. Learning the mood swing. A person is introduced to alcohol (in some cultures this can happen at a relatively young age), and the person enjoys the happy feeling it produces. At this stage, there is no emotional cost.

2. Seeking the mood swing. A person will drink to regain that feeling of euphoria experienced in phase 1; the drinking will increase as more intoxication is required to achieve the same effect. Again at this stage, there are no significant consequences.

3. At the third stage there are physical and social consequences, i.e., hangovers, family problems, work problems, etc. A person will continue to drink excessively, disregarding the problems.

4. The fourth stage can be detrimental, as Johnson cites it as a risk for premature death. As a person now drinks to feel normal, they block out the feelings of overwhelming guilt, remorse, anxiety, and shame they experience when sober.

Milam & Ketcham's Physical Deterioration Stages

Other theorists such as Milam & Ketcham (1983) focus on the physical deterioration that alcohol consumption causes. They describe the process in three stages:

1. Adaptive stage – The person will not experience any negative symptoms, and they believe they have the capacity for drinking alcohol without problems. Physiological changes are happening with the increase in tolerance, but this will not be noticeable to the drinker or others.

2. Dependent stage – At this stage, symptoms build up gradually. Hangover symptoms from excessive drinking may be confused with withdrawal symptoms. Many addicts will maintain their drinking to avoid withdrawal sickness, drinking small amounts frequently. They will try to hide their drinking problem from others and will avoid gross intoxication.

3. Deterioration stage – Various organs are damaged due to long-term drinking. Medical treatment in a rehabilitation center will be required; otherwise, the pathological changes will cause death.

DSM and ICD

In psychology and psychiatry, the DSM is the most common global standard, while in medicine, the standard is ICD. The terms they recommend are similar but not identical.

Organization	Preferred term(s)	Definition
APA's DSM-IV	"alcohol abuse" and "alcohol dependence"	• alcohol abuse = repeated use despite recurrent adverse consequences. • alcohol dependence = *alcohol abuse* combined with tolerance, withdrawal, and an uncontrollable drive to drink. The term "alcoholism" was split into "alcohol abuse" and "alcohol dependence" in 1980's DSM-III, and in 1987's DSM-III-R behavioral symptoms were moved from "abuse" to "dependence". It has been suggested that DSM-V merge alcohol abuse and alcohol dependence into a single new entry, named "alcohol-use disorder".
WHO's ICD-10	"alcohol harmful use" and "alcohol dependence syndrome"	Definitions are similar to that of the DSM-IV. The World Health Organisation uses the term "alcohol dependence syndrome" rather than alcoholism. The concept of "harmful use" (as opposed to "abuse") was introduced in 1992's ICD-10 to minimize underreporting of damage in the absence of dependence. The term "alcoholism" was removed from ICD between ICD-8/ICDA-8 and ICD-9.

The DSM-IV diagnosis of alcohol dependence represents one approach to the definition of alcoholism. In part, this is to assist in the development of research protocols in which findings can be compared to one another. According to the DSM-IV, an alcohol dependence diagnosis is: "maladaptive alcohol use with clinically significant impairment as manifested by at least three of the following within any one-year period: tolerance; withdrawal; taken in greater amounts or over longer time course than intended; desire or unsuccessful attempts to cut down or control use; great deal of time spent obtaining, using, or recovering from use; social, occupational, or recreational activities given up or reduced; continued use despite knowledge of physical or psychological sequelae." Despite the imprecision inherent in the term, there have been attempts to define how the word *alcoholism* should be interpreted when encountered. In 1992, it was defined by the National Council on Alcoholism and Drug Dependence (NCADD) and ASAM as "a primary, chronic disease characterized by impaired control over drinking, preoccupation with the drug alcohol, use of alcohol despite adverse consequences, and distortions in thinking." MeSH has had an entry for "alcoholism" since 1999, and references the 1992 definition.

AA describes alcoholism as an illness that involves a physical allergy (where "allergy" has a different meaning than that used in modern medicine.) and a mental obsession. The doctor and addiction specialist Dr. William D. Silkworth M.D. writes on behalf of AA that "Alcoholics suffer from a "(physical) craving beyond mental control". A 1960 study by E. Morton Jellinek is considered the foundation of the modern disease theory of alcoholism. Jellinek's definition restricted the use of the word *alcoholism* to those showing a particular natural history. The modern medical definition of *alcoholism* has been revised numerous times since then. The American Medical Association uses the word alcoholism to refer to a particular chronic primary disease.

Social Barriers

Attitudes and social stereotypes can create barriers to the detection and treatment of alcohol abuse. This is more of a barrier for women than men. Fear of stigmatization may lead women to deny that they are suffering from a medical condition, to hide their drinking, and to drink alone. This pattern, in turn, leads family, physicians, and others to be less likely to suspect that a woman they know is an alcoholic. In contrast, reduced fear of stigma may lead men to admit that they are suffering from a medical condition, to display their drinking publicly, and to drink in groups. This pattern, in turn, leads family, physicians, and others to be more likely to suspect that a man they know is an alcoholic.

Screening

Several tools may be used to detect a loss of control of alcohol use. These tools are mostly self-reports in questionnaire form. Another common theme is a score or tally that sums up the general severity of alcohol use.

The CAGE questionnaire, named for its four questions, is one such example that may be used to screen patients quickly in a doctor's office.

Two "yes" responses indicate that the respondent should be investigated further.

The questionnaire asks the following questions:

1. Have you ever felt you needed to Cut down on your drinking?
2. Have people Annoyed you by criticizing your drinking?
3. Have you ever felt Guilty about drinking?
4. Have you ever felt you needed a drink first thing in the morning (Eye-opener) to steady your nerves or to get rid of a hangover?

   The CAGE questionnaire has demonstrated a high effectiveness in detecting alcohol-related problems; however, it has limitations in people with less severe alcohol-related problems, white women and college students.

Other tests are sometimes used for the detection of alcohol dependence, such as the Alcohol Dependence Data Questionnaire, which is a more sensitive diagnostic test than the CAGE questionnaire. It helps distinguish a diagnosis of alcohol dependence from one of heavy alcohol use. The Michigan Alcohol Screening Test (MAST) is a screening tool for alcoholism widely used by courts to determine the appropriate sentencing for people convicted of alcohol-related offenses, driving under the influence being the most common. The Alcohol Use Disorders Identification Test (AUDIT), a screening questionnaire developed by the World Health Organization, is unique in that it has been validated in six countries and is used internationally. Like the CAGE questionnaire, it uses a simple set of questions – a high score earning a deeper investigation. The Paddington Alcohol Test (PAT) was designed to screen for alcohol-related problems amongst those attending Accident and Emergency departments. It concords well with the AUDIT questionnaire but is administered in a fifth of the time. Certain blood tests may also indicate possible alcoholism.

Genetic Predisposition Testing

Psychiatric geneticists John I. Nurnberger, Jr., and Laura Jean Bierut suggest that alcoholism does not have a single cause—including genetic—but that genes do play an important role "by affecting processes in the body and brain that interact with one another and with an individual's life experiences to produce protection or susceptibility". They also report that fewer than a dozen alcoholism-related genes have been identified, but that more likely await discovery. At least one genetic test exists for an allele that is correlated to alcoholism and opiate addiction. Human dopamine receptor genes have a detectable variation referred to as the DRD2 TaqI polymorphism. Those who possess the A1 allele (variation) of this polymorphism have a small but significant tendency towards addiction to opiates and endorphin-releasing drugs like alcohol. Although this allele is slightly more common in alcoholics and opiate addicts, it is not by itself an adequate predictor of alcoholism, and some researchers argue that evidence for DRD2 is contradictory.

Urine and Blood Tests

There are reliable tests for the actual use of alcohol, one common test being that of blood alcohol content (BAC). These tests do not differentiate alcoholics from non-alcoholics; however, long-term heavy drinking does have a few recognizable effects on the body, including:

- Macrocytosis (enlarged MCV)
- Elevated GGT
- Moderate elevation of AST and ALT and an AST: ALT ratio of 2:1
- High carbohydrate deficient transferrin (CDT)

With regard to alcoholism, BAC is useful to judge alcohol tolerance, which in turn is a sign of alcoholism.

However, none of these blood tests for biological markers is as sensitive as screening questionnaires.

Prevention

The World Health Organization, the European Union and other regional bodies, national governments and parliaments have formed alcohol policies in order to reduce the harm of alcoholism. Targeting adolescents and young adults is regarded as an important step to reduce the harm of alcohol abuse. Increasing the age at which licit drugs of abuse such as alcohol can be purchased, the banning or restricting advertising of alcohol has been recommended as additional ways of reducing the harm of alcohol dependence and abuse. Credible, evidence based educational campaigns in the mass media about the consequences of alcohol abuse have been recommended. Guidelines for parents to prevent alcohol abuse amongst adolescents, and for helping young people with mental health problems have also been suggested.

Management

Treatments are varied because there are multiple perspectives of alcoholism. Those who approach alcoholism as a medical condition or disease recommend differing treatments from, for instance, those who approach the condition as one of social choice. Most treatments focus on helping people discontinue their alcohol intake, followed up with life training and/or social support to help them resist a return to alcohol use. Since alcoholism involves multiple factors which encourage a person to continue drinking, they must all be addressed to successfully prevent a relapse. An example of this kind of treatment is detoxification followed by a combination of supportive therapy, attendance at self-help groups, and ongoing development of coping mechanisms. The treatment community for alcoholism typically supports an abstinence-based zero tolerance approach; however, some prefer a harm-reduction approach.

Detoxification

Alcohol detoxification or 'detox' for alcoholics is an abrupt stop of alcohol drinking coupled with the substitution of drugs, such as benzodiazepines, that have similar effects to prevent alcohol withdrawal. Individuals who are only at risk of mild to moderate withdrawal symptoms can be detoxified as outpatients. Individuals at risk of a severe withdrawal syndrome as well as those who have significant or acute comorbid conditions are generally treated as inpatients. Detoxification does not actually treat alcoholism, and it is necessary to follow up detoxification with an appropriate treatment program for alcohol dependence or abuse to reduce the risk of relapse. Some symptoms of alcohol withdrawal such as depressed mood and anxiety typically take weeks or months to abate while other symptoms persist longer due to persisting neuroadaptations. Alcoholism has serious adverse effects on brain function; on average it takes one year of abstinence to recover from the cognitive deficits incurred by chronic alcohol abuse.

Psychological

Various forms of group therapy or psychotherapy can be used to deal with underlying psychological issues that are related to alcohol addiction, as well as provide relapse prevention skills. The mutual-help group-counseling approach is one of the most common ways of helping alcoholics maintain sobriety. Alcoholics Anonymous was one of the first organizations formed to provide mutual, nonprofessional counseling, and it is still the largest. Others include LifeRing Secular Recovery, SMART Recovery, Women For Sobriety, and Secular Organizations for Sobriety. Rationing and moderation programs such as Moderation Management and DrinkWise do not mandate complete abstinence. While most alcoholics are unable to limit their drinking in this way, some return to moderate drinking. A 2002 US study by the National Institute on Alcohol Abuse and Alcoholism (NIAAA) showed that 17.7 percent of individuals diagnosed as alcohol dependent more than one year prior returned to low-risk drinking. This group, however, showed fewer initial symptoms of dependency. A follow-up study, using the same subjects that were judged to be in remission in 2001–2002, examined the rates of return to problem drinking in 2004–2005. The study found abstinence from alcohol was the most stable form of remission for recovering alcoholics. A long-term (60 year) follow-up of two groups of alcoholic men concluded that "return to controlled drinking rarely persisted for much more than a decade without relapse or evolution into abstinence."

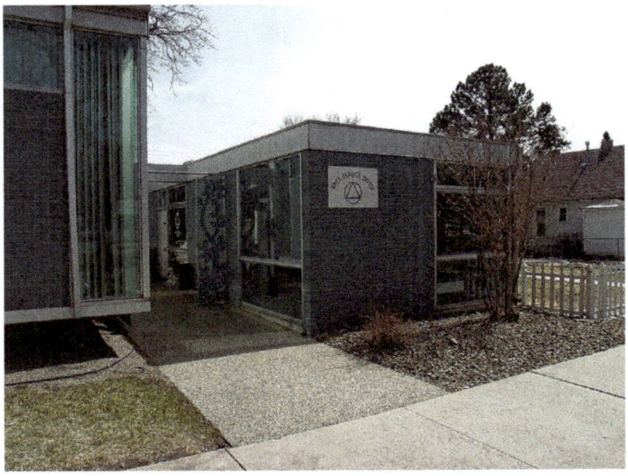

A regional service center for Alcoholics Anonymous

Medications

In the United States there are four approved medications for alcoholism: disulfiram, two forms of naltrexone, and acamprosate. Several other drugs are also used and many are under investigation.

- Benzodiazepines, while useful in the management of acute alcohol withdrawal, if used long-term can cause a worse outcome in alcoholism. Alcoholics on chronic benzodiazepines have a lower rate of achieving abstinence from alcohol than those not taking benzodiazepines. This class of drugs is commonly prescribed to alcoholics for insomnia or anxiety management. Initiating prescriptions of benzodiazepines or sedative-hypnotics in individuals in recovery has a high rate of relapse with one author reporting more than a quarter of people relapsed after being prescribed sedative-hypnotics. Those who are long-term users of benzodiazepines should not be withdrawn rapidly, as severe anxiety and panic may develop, which are known risk factors for relapse into alcohol abuse. Taper regimes of 6–12 months have been found to be the most successful, with reduced intensity of withdrawal.

- Acamprosate may stabilise the brain chemistry that is altered due to alcohol dependence via antagonising the actions of glutamate, a neurotransmitter which is hyperactive in the post-withdrawal phase. By reducing excessive NMDA activity which occurs at the onset of alcohol withdrawal, acamprosate can reduce or prevent alcohol withdrawal related neurotoxicity. Acamprosate reduces the risk of relapse amongst alcohol dependent persons.
- Disulfiram (Antabuse) prevents the elimination of acetaldehyde, a chemical the body produces when breaking down ethanol. Acetaldehyde itself is the cause of many hangover symptoms from alcohol use. The overall effect is severe discomfort when alcohol is ingested: an extremely fast-acting and long-lasting uncomfortable hangover. This discourages an alcoholic from drinking in significant amounts while they take the medicine.
- Naltrexone is a competitive antagonist for opioid receptors, effectively blocking the effects of endorphins and opioids. Naltrexone is used to decrease cravings for alcohol and encourage abstinence. Alcohol causes the body to release endorphins, which in turn release dopamine and activate the reward pathways; hence when naltrexone is in the body there is a reduction in the pleasurable effects from consuming alcohol. Evidence supports a reduced risk of relapse among alcohol dependent persons and a decrease in excessive drinking. Nalmefene also appears effective and works by a similar manner.
- Calcium carbimide works in the same way as disulfiram; it has an advantage in that the occasional adverse effects of disulfiram, hepatotoxicity and drowsiness, do not occur with calcium carbimide.

The Sinclair method is a method of using naltrexone or another opioid antagonists to treat alcoholism by having the person take the medication about an hour before they drink alcohol, and only then. The medication blocks the positive reinforcement effects of ethanol and hopefully allows the person to stop drinking or drink less.

Evidence does not support the use of selective serotonin reuptake inhibitors (SSRIs), tricyclic antidepressants (TCAs), antipsychotics, or gabapentin.

Dual Addictions and Dependences

Alcoholics may also require treatment for other psychotropic drug addictions and drug dependences. The most common dual dependence syndrome with alcohol dependence is benzodiazepine dependence, with studies showing 10–20 percent of alcohol-dependent individuals had problems of dependence and/or misuse problems of benzodiazepine drugs such as valium or clonazopam. These drugs are, like alcohol, depressants. Benzodiazepines may be used legally, if they are prescribed by doctors for anxiety problems or other mood disorders, or they may be purchased as illegal drugs "on the street" through illicit channels. Benzodiazepine use increases cravings for alcohol and the volume of alcohol consumed by problem drinkers. Benzodiazepine dependency requires careful reduction in dosage to avoid benzodiazepine withdrawal syndrome and other health consequences. Dependence on other sedative-hypnotics such as zolpidem and zopiclone as well as opiates and illegal drugs is common in alcoholics. Alcohol itself is a sedative-hypnotic and is cross-tolerant with other sedative-hypnotics such as barbiturates, benzodiazepines and nonbenzodiazepines. Dependence upon and withdrawal from sedative-hypnotics can be medically severe and, as with alcohol withdrawal, there is a risk of psychosis or seizures if not managed properly.

Epidemiology

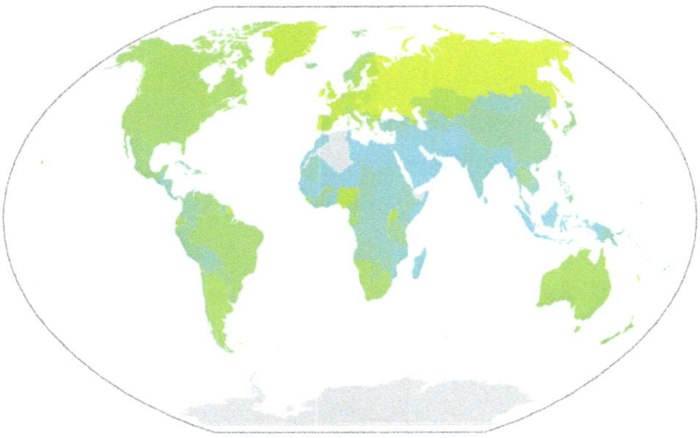

Total recorded yearly alcohol per capita consumption (15+), in litres of pure alcohol

The World Health Organization estimates that as of 2010 there are 208 million people with alcoholism worldwide (4.1% of the population over 15 years of age). Substance use disorders are a major public health problem facing many countries. "The most common substance of abuse/dependence in patients presenting for treatment is alcohol." In the United Kingdom, the number of 'dependent drinkers' was calculated as over 2.8 million in 2001. About 12% of American adults have had an alcohol dependence problem at some time in their life. In the United States and Western Europe, 10 to 20 percent of men and 5 to 10 percent of women at some point in their lives will meet criteria for alcoholism. Estonia had the highest death rate from alcohol in Europe in 2015 at 8.8 per 100,000 population.

Within the medical and scientific communities, there is a broad consensus regarding alcoholism as a disease state. For example, the American Medical Association considers alcohol a drug and states that "drug addiction is a chronic, relapsing brain disease characterized by compulsive drug seeking and use despite often devastating consequences. It results from a complex interplay of biological vulnerability, environmental exposure, and developmental factors (e.g., stage of brain maturity)." Alcoholism has a higher prevalence among men, though, in recent decades, the proportion of female alcoholics has increased. Current evidence indicates that in both men and women, alcoholism is 50–60 percent genetically determined, leaving 40–50 percent for environmental influences. Most alcoholics develop alcoholism during adolescence or young adulthood. 31 percent of college students show signs of alcohol abuse, while six percent are dependent on alcohol. Under the DSM's new definition of alcoholics, that means about 37 percent of college students may meet the criteria.

Prognosis

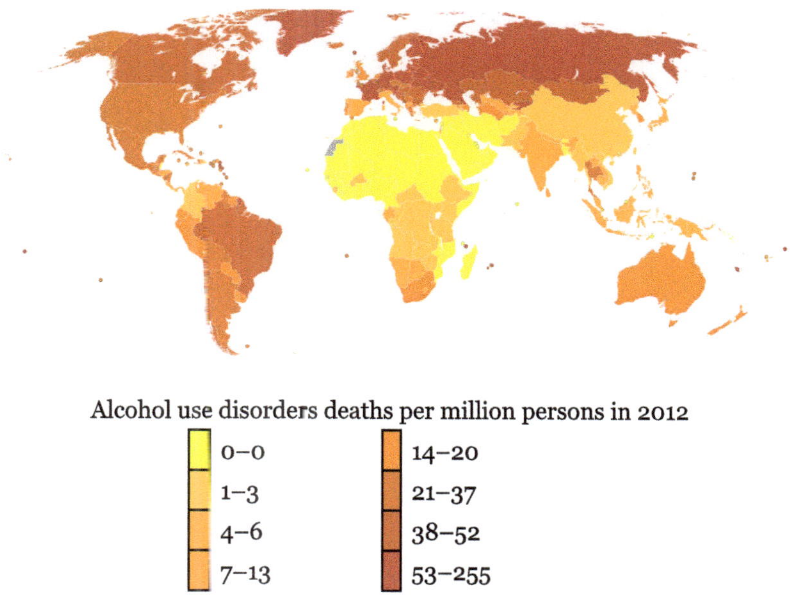

Alcoholism often reduces a person's life expectancy by around ten years. The most common cause of death in alcoholics is from cardiovascular complications. There is a high rate of suicide in chronic alcoholics, which increases the longer a person drinks. Approximately 3–15 percent of alcoholics commit suicide, and research has found that over 50 percent of all suicides are associated with alcohol or drug dependence. This is believed to be due to alcohol causing physiological distortion of brain chemistry, as well as social isolation. Suicide is also very common in adolescent alcohol abusers, with 25 percent of suicides in adolescents being related to alcohol abuse. Among those with alcohol dependence after one year, some met the criteria for low-risk drinking, even though only 25.5 percent of the group received any treatment, with the breakdown as follows: 25 percent were found to be still dependent, 27.3 percent were in partial remission (some symptoms persist), 11.8 percent asymptomatic drinkers (consumption increases chances of relapse) and 35.9 percent were fully recovered—made up of 17.7

percent low-risk drinkers plus 18.2 percent abstainers. In contrast, however, the results of a long-term (60-year) follow-up of two groups of alcoholic men indicated that "return to controlled drinking rarely persisted for much more than a decade without relapse or evolution into abstinence." There was also "return-to-controlled drinking, as reported in short-term studies, is often a mirage."

History

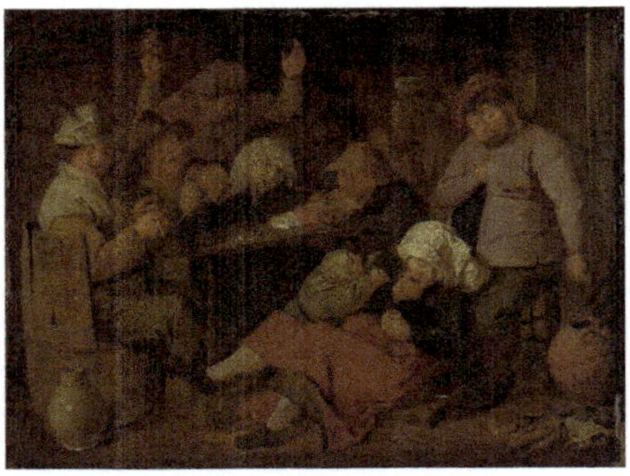

Adriaen Brouwer, *Inn with Drunken Peasants*, 1620s

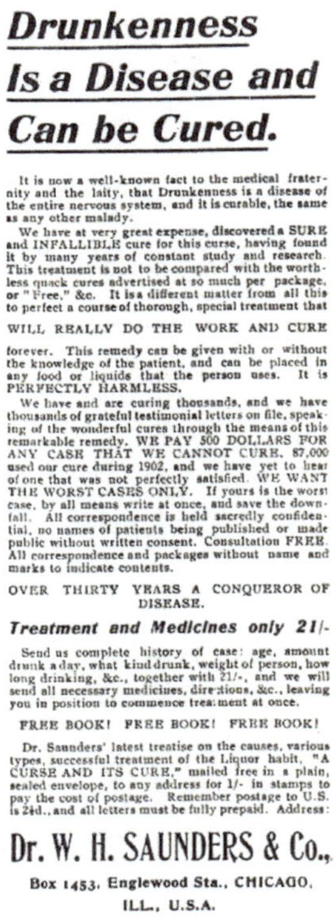

1904 advertisement describing alcoholism as a disease

Historically the name "dipsomania" was coined by German physician C. W. Hufeland in 1819 before it was superseded by "alcoholism". That term now has a more specific meaning. The term "alcoholism" was first used in 1849 by the Swedish physician Magnus Huss to describe the systematic adverse effects of alcohol. Alcohol has a long history of use and misuse throughout recorded history. Biblical, Egyptian and Babylonian sources record the history of abuse and dependence on alcohol. In some ancient cultures alcohol was worshiped and in others, its abuse was condemned. Excessive alcohol misuse and drunkenness were recognized as causing social problems even thousands of years ago. However, the defining of habitual drunkenness as it was then known as and its adverse consequences were not well established medically until the 18th century. In 1647 a Greek monk named Agapios was the first to document that chronic alcohol misuse was associated with toxicity to the nervous system and body which resulted in a range of medical disorders such as seizures, paralysis, and internal bleeding. In 1920 the effects of alcohol abuse and chronic drunkenness led to the failed prohibition of alcohol being considered and eventually enforced briefly in America. In 2005 alcohol dependence and abuse was estimated to cost the US economy approximately 220 billion dollars per year, more than cancer and obesity.

Society and Culture

The various health problems associated with long-term alcohol consumption are generally perceived as detrimental to society, for example, money due to lost labor-hours, medical costs due to injuries due to drunkenness and organ damage from long-term use, and secondary treatment costs, such as the costs of rehabilitation facilities and detoxification centers. Alcohol use is a major contributing factor for head injuries, motor vehicle accidents (due to drunk driving), domestic violence, and assaults. Beyond the financial costs that alcohol consumption imposes, there are also significant social costs to both the alcoholic and their family and friends. For instance, alcohol consumption by a pregnant woman can lead to fetal alcohol syndrome, an incurable and damaging condition. Estimates of the economic costs of alcohol abuse, collected by the World Health Organization, vary from one to six percent of a country's GDP. One Australian estimate pegged alcohol's social costs at 24% of all drug abuse costs; a similar Canadian study concluded alcohol's share was 41%. One study quantified the cost to the UK of *all* forms of alcohol misuse in 2001 as £18.5–20 billion. All economic costs in the United States in 2006 have been estimated at $223.5 billion.

Stereotypes of alcoholics are often found in fiction and popular culture. The "town drunk" is a stock character in Western popular culture. Stereotypes of drunkenness may be based on racism or xenophobia, as in the fictional depiction of the Irish as heavy drinkers. Studies by social psychologists Stivers and Greeley attempt to document the perceived prevalence of high alcohol consumption amongst the Irish in America. Alcohol consumption is relatively similar between many European cultures, the United States, and Australia. In Asian countries that have a high gross domestic product, there is heightened drinking compared to other Asian countries, but it is nowhere near as high as it is in other countries like the United States. It is also inversely seen, with countries that have very low gross domestic product showing high alcohol consumption. In a study done on Korean immigrants in Canada, they reported alcohol was even an integral part of their meal, and is the only time solo drinking should occur. They also believe alcohol is necessary at any social event as it helps conversations start.

Caucasians have a much lower abstinence rate (11.8%) and much higher tolerance to symptoms (3.4±2.45 drinks) of alcohol than Chinese (33.4% and 2.2±1.78 drinks respectively). Also, the more acculturation there is between cultures, the more influenced the culture is to adopt Caucasians drinking practices. Peyote, a psychoactive agent, has even shown promise in treating alcoholism. Alcohol had actually replaced peyote as Native Americans' psychoactive agent of choice in rituals when peyote was outlawed.

Research

Topiramate

Topiramate, a derivative of the naturally occurring sugar monosaccharide D-fructose, has been found effective in helping alcoholics quit or cut back on the amount they drink. Evidence suggests that topiramate antagonizes excitatory glutamate receptors, inhibits dopamine release, and enhances inhibitory gamma-aminobutyric acid function. A 2008 review of the effectiveness of topiramate concluded that the results of published trials are promising, however, as of 2008, data was insufficient to support using topiramate in conjunction with brief weekly compliance counseling as a first-line agent for alcohol dependence. A 2010 review found that topiramate may be superior to existing alcohol pharmacotherapeutic options. Topiramate effectively reduces craving and alcohol withdrawal severity as well as improving quality-of-life-ratings.

Baclofen

Baclofen, a GABAB receptor agonist, is under study for the treatment of alcoholism. A 2015 systematic review concluded that there is insufficient evidence for the use of baclofen for withdrawal symptoms in alcoholism. There is tentative data supporting baclofen in alcohol dependence however further trials are needed as of 2013.

Ondansetron

Ondansetron, a 5HT3 antagonist, appears to have promise as a treatment.

Amphetamine

Amphetamine (contracted from alphamethylphenethylamine) is a potent central nervous system (CNS) stimulant that is used in the treatment of attention deficit hyperactivity disorder (ADHD), narcolepsy, and obesity. Amphetamine was discovered in

1887 and exists as two enantiomers: levoamphetamine and dextroamphetamine. *Amphetamine* properly refers to a specific chemical, the racemic free base, which is equal parts of the two enantiomers, levoamphetamine and dextroamphetamine, in their pure amine forms. The term is frequently used informally to refer to any combination of the enantiomers, or to either of them alone. Historically, it has been used to treat nasal congestion and depression. Amphetamine is also used as an athletic performance enhancer and cognitive enhancer, and recreationally as an aphrodisiac and euphoriant. It is a prescription drug in many countries, and unauthorized possession and distribution of amphetamine are often tightly controlled due to the significant health risks associated with recreational use.

The first amphetamine pharmaceutical was Benzedrine, a brand which was used to treat a variety of conditions. Currently, pharmaceutical amphetamine is prescribed as racemic amphetamine, Adderall, dextroamphetamine, or the inactive prodrug lisdexamfetamine. Amphetamine, through activation of a trace amine receptor, increases monoamine and excitatory neurotransmitter activity in the brain, with its most pronounced effects targeting the catecholamine neurotransmitters norepinephrine and dopamine.

At therapeutic doses, amphetamine causes emotional and cognitive effects such as euphoria, change in desire for sex, increased wakefulness, and improved cognitive control. It induces physical effects such as decreased reaction time, fatigue resistance, and increased muscle strength. Larger doses of amphetamine may impair cognitive function and induce rapid muscle breakdown. Drug addiction is a serious risk with large recreational doses but is unlikely to arise from typical long-term medical use at therapeutic doses. Very high doses can result in psychosis (e.g., delusions and paranoia) which rarely occurs at therapeutic doses even during long-term use. Recreational doses are generally much larger than prescribed therapeutic doses and carry a far greater risk of serious side effects.

Amphetamine belongs to the phenethylamine class. It is also the parent compound of its own structural class, the substituted amphetamines, which includes prominent substances such as bupropion, cathinone, MDMA, and methamphetamine. As a member of the phenethylamine class, amphetamine is also chemically related to the naturally occurring trace amine neuromodulators, specifically phenethylamine and *N*-methylphenethylamine, both of which are produced within the human body. Phenethylamine is the parent compound of amphetamine, while *N*-methylphenethylamine is a positional isomer of amphetamine that differs only in the placement of the methyl group.

Uses

Medical

Amphetamine is used to treat attention deficit hyperactivity disorder (ADHD), narcolepsy (a sleep disorder), and obesity, and is sometimes prescribed off-label for its past medical indications, such as depression. Long-term amphetamine exposure at sufficiently high doses in some animal species is known to produce abnormal dopamine system development or nerve damage, but, in humans with ADHD, pharmaceutical amphetamines appear to improve brain development and nerve growth. Reviews of magnetic resonance imaging (MRI) studies suggest that long-term treatment with amphetamine decreases abnormalities in brain structure and function found in subjects with ADHD, and improves function in several parts of the brain, such as the right caudate nucleus of the basal ganglia.

Reviews of clinical stimulant research have established the safety and effectiveness of long-term continuous amphetamine use for the treatment of ADHD. Randomized controlled trials of continuous stimulant therapy for the treatment of ADHD spanning two years have demonstrated treatment effectiveness and safety. Two reviews have indicated that long-term continuous stimulant therapy for ADHD is effective for reducing the core symptoms of ADHD (i.e., hyperactivity, inattention, and impulsivity), enhancing quality of life and academic achievement, and producing improvements in a large number of functional outcomes across nine outcome categories related to academics, antisocial behavior, driving, non-medicinal drug use, obesity, occupation, self-esteem, service use (i.e., academic, occupational, health, financial, and legal services), and social function. One review highlighted a nine-month randomized controlled trial in children with ADHD that found an average increase of 4.5 IQ points, continued increases in attention, and continued decreases in disruptive behaviors and hyperactivity. Another review indicated that, based upon the longest follow-up studies conducted to date, lifetime stimulant therapy that begins during childhood is continuously effective for controlling ADHD symptoms and reduces the risk of developing a substance use disorder as an adult.

Current models of ADHD suggest that it is associated with functional impairments in some of the brain's neurotransmitter systems; these functional impairments involve impaired dopamine neurotransmission in the mesocorticolimbic projection and norepinephrine neurotransmission in the noradrenergic projections from the locus coeruleus to the prefrontal cortex. Psychostimulants like methylphenidate and amphetamine are effective in treating ADHD because they increase neurotransmitter activity in these systems. Approximately 80% of those who use these stimulants see improvements in ADHD symptoms. Children with ADHD who use stimulant medications generally have better relationships with peers and family members, perform better in school, are less distractible and impulsive, and have longer attention spans. The Cochrane Collaboration's reviews on the treatment of ADHD in children, adolescents, and adults with pharmaceutical amphetamines stated that while these drugs improve short-term symptoms, they have higher discontinuation rates than non-stimulant medications due to their adverse side effects. A Cochrane Collaboration review on the treatment of ADHD in children with tic disorders such as Tourette syndrome indicated that stimulants in general do not make tics worse, but high doses of dextroamphetamine could exacerbate tics in some individuals.

Enhancing Performance

Cognitive

In 2015, a systematic review and a meta-analysis of high quality clinical trials found that, when used at low (therapeutic) doses, amphetamine produces modest yet unambiguous improvements in cognition, including working memory, long-term episodic memory, inhibitory control, and some aspects of attention, in normal healthy adults; these cognition-enhancing effects of amphetamine are known to be partially mediated through the indirect activation of both dopamine receptor D_1 and adrenoceptor α_2 in the prefrontal cortex. A systematic review from 2014 found that low doses of amphetamine also improve memory consolidation, in turn leading to improved recall of information. Therapeutic doses of amphetamine also enhance cortical network efficiency, an effect which mediates improvements in working memory in all individuals. Amphetamine and other ADHD stimulants also improve task saliency (motivation to perform a task) and increase arousal (wakefulness), in turn promoting goal-directed behavior. Stimulants such as amphetamine can improve performance on difficult and boring tasks and are used by some students as a study and test-taking aid. Based upon studies of self-reported illicit stimulant use, 5–35% of college students use diverted ADHD stimulants, which are primarily used for performance enhancement rather than as recreational drugs. However, high amphetamine doses that are above the therapeutic range can interfere with working memory and other aspects of cognitive control.

Physical

Amphetamine is used by some athletes for its psychological and athletic performance-enhancing effects, such as increased endurance and alertness; however, non-medical amphetamine use is prohibited at sporting events that are regulated by collegiate, national, and international anti-doping agencies. In healthy people at oral therapeutic doses, amphetamine has been shown to increase muscle strength, acceleration, athletic performance in anaerobic conditions, and endurance (i.e., it delays the onset of fatigue), while improving reaction time. Amphetamine improves endurance and reaction time primarily through reuptake inhibition and effluxion of dopamine in the central nervous system. Amphetamine and other dopaminergic drugs also increase power output at fixed levels of perceived exertion by overriding a "safety switch" that allows the core temperature limit to increase in order to access a reserve capacity that is normally off-limits. At therapeutic doses, the adverse effects of amphetamine do not impede athletic performance; however, at much higher doses, amphetamine can induce effects that severely impair performance, such as rapid muscle breakdown and elevated body temperature.

Contraindications

According to the International Programme on Chemical Safety (IPCS) and United States Food and Drug Administration (USFDA), amphetamine is contraindicated in people with a history of drug abuse, cardiovascular disease, severe agitation, or severe anxiety. It is also contraindicated in people currently experiencing arteriosclerosis (hardening of the arteries), glaucoma (increased eye pressure), hyperthyroidism (excessive production of thyroid hormone), or moderate to severe hypertension. People who have experienced allergic reactions to other stimulants in the past or who are taking monoamine oxidase inhibitors (MAOIs) are advised not to take amphetamine, although safe concurrent use of amphetamine and monoamine oxidase inhibitors has been documented. These agencies also state that anyone with anorexia nervosa, bipolar disorder, depression, hypertension, liver or kidney problems, mania, psychosis, Raynaud's phenomenon, seizures, thyroid problems, tics, or Tourette syndrome should monitor their symptoms while taking amphetamine. Evidence from human studies indicates that therapeutic amphetamine use does not cause developmental abnormalities in the fetus or newborns (i.e., it is not a human teratogen), but amphetamine abuse does pose risks to the fetus. Amphetamine has also been shown to pass into breast milk, so the IPCS and USFDA advise mothers to avoid breastfeeding when using it. Due to the potential for reversible growth impairments, the USFDA advises monitoring the height and weight of children and adolescents prescribed an amphetamine pharmaceutical.

Side Effects

The side effects of amphetamine are varied, and the amount of amphetamine used is the primary factor in determining the likelihood and severity of side effects. Amphetamine products such as Adderall, Dexedrine, and their generic equivalents are currently approved by the USFDA for long-term therapeutic use. Recreational use of amphetamine generally involves much larger doses, which have a greater risk of serious side effects than dosages used for therapeutic reasons.

Physical

At normal therapeutic doses, the physical side effects of amphetamine vary widely by age and from person to person. Cardiovascular side effects can include hypertension or hypotension from a vasovagal response, Raynaud's phenomenon (reduced blood flow to the hands and feet), and tachycardia (increased heart rate). Sexual side effects in males may include erectile dysfunction, frequent erections, or prolonged erections. Abdominal side effects may include abdominal pain, appetite loss, nausea, and weight loss. Other potential side effects include blurred vision, dry mouth, excessive grinding of the teeth, nosebleed, profuse sweating, rhinitis medicamentosa (drug-induced nasal congestion), reduced seizure threshold, and tics (a type of movement disorder). Dangerous physical side effects are rare at typical pharmaceutical doses.

Amphetamine stimulates the medullary respiratory centers, producing faster and deeper breaths. In a normal person at therapeutic doses, this effect is usually not noticeable, but when respiration is already compromised, it may be evident. Amphetamine also induces contraction in the urinary bladder sphincter, the muscle which controls urination, which can result in difficulty urinating. This effect can be useful in treating bed wetting and loss of bladder control. The effects of amphetamine on the gastrointestinal tract are unpredictable. If intestinal activity is high, amphetamine may reduce gastrointestinal motility (the rate at which content moves through the digestive system); however, amphetamine may increase motility when the smooth muscle of the tract is relaxed. Amphetamine also has a slight analgesic effect and can enhance the pain relieving effects of opioids.

USFDA-commissioned studies from 2011 indicate that in children, young adults, and adults there is no association between serious adverse cardiovascular events (sudden death, heart attack, and stroke) and the medical use of amphetamine or other ADHD stimulants. However, amphetamine pharmaceuticals are contraindicated in individuals with cardiovascular disease.

Psychological

At normal therapeutic doses, the most common psychological side effects of amphetamine include increased alertness, apprehension, concentration, initiative, self-confidence, and sociability, mood swings (elated mood followed by mildly depressed mood), insomnia or wakefulness, and decreased sense of fatigue. Less common side effects include anxiety, change in libido, grandiosity, irritability, repetitive or obsessive behaviors, and restlessness; these effects depend on the user's personality and current mental state. Amphetamine psychosis (e.g., delusions and paranoia) can occur in heavy users. Although very rare, this psychosis can also occur at therapeutic doses during long-term therapy. According to the USFDA, "there is no systematic evidence" that stimulants produce aggressive behavior or hostility.

Amphetamine has also been shown to produce a conditioned place preference in humans taking therapeutic doses, meaning that individuals acquire a preference for spending time in places where they have previously used amphetamine.

Overdose

An amphetamine overdose can lead to many different symptoms, but is rarely fatal with appropriate care. The severity of overdose symptoms increases with dosage and decreases with drug tolerance to amphetamine. Tolerant individuals have been known to take as much as 5 grams of amphetamine in a day, which is roughly 100 times the maximum daily therapeutic dose. Symptoms of a moderate and extremely large overdose are listed below; fatal amphetamine poisoning usually also involves convulsions and coma. In 2013, overdose on amphetamine, methamphetamine, and other compounds implicated in an "amphetamine use disorder" resulted in an estimated 3,788 deaths worldwide (3,425–4,145 deaths, 95% confidence).

Pathological overactivation of the mesolimbic pathway, a dopamine pathway that connects the ventral tegmental area to the nucleus accumbens, plays a central role in amphetamine addiction. Individuals who frequently overdose on amphetamine during recreational use have a high risk of developing an amphetamine addiction, since repeated overdoses gradually increase the level of accumbal ΔFosB, a "molecular switch" and "master control protein" for addiction. Once nucleus accumbens ΔFosB is sufficiently overexpressed, it begins to increase the severity of addictive behavior (i.e., compulsive drug-seeking) with further increases in its expression. While there are currently no effective drugs for treating amphetamine addiction, regularly engaging in sustained aerobic exercise appears to reduce the risk of developing such an addiction. Sustained aerobic exercise on a regular basis also appears to be an effective treatment for amphetamine addiction; exercise therapy improves clinical treatment outcomes and may be used as a combination therapy with cognitive behavioral therapy, which is currently the best clinical treatment available.

Overdose Symptoms by System		
System	**Minor or Moderate Overdose**	**Severe Overdose**
Cardiovascular	• Abnormal heartbeat • High or low blood pressure	• Cardiogenic shock (heart not pumping enough blood) • Cerebral hemorrhage (bleeding in the brain) • Circulatory collapse (partial or complete failure of the circulatory system)
Central nervous system	• Confusion • Abnormally fast reflexes • Severe agitation • Tremor (involuntary muscle twitching)	• Acute amphetamine psychosis (e.g., delusions and paranoia) • Compulsive and repetitive movement • Serotonin syndrome (excessive serotonergic nerve activity) • Sympathomimetic toxidrome (excessive adrenergic nerve activity)
Musculoskeletal	• Muscle pain	• Rhabdomyolysis (rapid muscle breakdown)
Respiratory	• Rapid breathing	• Pulmonary edema (fluid accumulation in the lungs) • Pulmonary hypertension (high blood pressure in the arteries of the lung) • Respiratory alkalosis (reduced blood CO_2)
Urinary	• Painful urination • Urinary retention (inability to urinate)	• No urine production • Kidney failure

Other	• Elevated body temperature • Mydriasis (dilated pupils)	• Elevated or low blood potassium • Hyperpyrexia (extremely elevated core body temperature) • Metabolic acidosis (excessively acidic bodily fluids)

Addiction

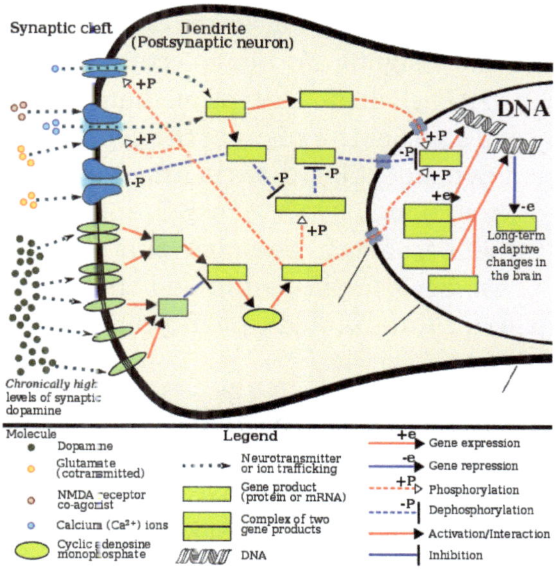

Signaling cascade in the nucleus accumbens that results in amphetamine addiction

This diagram depicts the signaling events in the brain's reward center that are induced by chronic high-dose exposure to psychostimulants that increase the concentration of synaptic dopamine, like amphetamine, methamphetamine, and phenethylamine. Following presynaptic dopamine and glutamate co-release by such psychostimulants, postsynaptic receptors for these neurotransmitters trigger internal signaling events through a cAMP-dependent pathway and a calcium-dependent pathway that ultimately result in increased CREB phosphorylation. Phosphorylated CREB increases levels of ΔFosB, which in turn represses the c-Fos gene with the help of corepressors; c-Fos repression acts as a molecular switch that enables the accumulation of ΔFosB in the neuron. A highly stable (phosphorylated) form of ΔFosB, one that persists in neurons for one or two months, slowly accumulates following repeated high-dose exposure to stimulants through this process. ΔFosB functions as "one of the master control proteins" that produces addiction-related structural changes in the brain, and upon sufficient accumulation, with the help of its downstream targets (e.g., nuclear factor kappa B), it induces an addictive state.

Addiction is a serious risk with heavy recreational amphetamine use but is unlikely to arise from typical long-term medical use at therapeutic doses. Drug tolerance develops rapidly in amphetamine abuse (i.e., a recreational amphetamine overdose), so periods of extended use require increasingly larger doses of the drug in order to achieve the same effect.

Biomolecular Mechanisms

Chronic use of amphetamine at excessive doses causes alterations in gene expression in the mesocorticolimbic projection, which arise through transcriptional and epigenetic mechanisms. The most important transcription factors that produce these alterations are ΔFosB, cAMP response element binding protein (CREB), and nuclear factor kappa B (NF-κB). ΔFosB is the most significant biomolecular mechanism in addiction because the overexpression of ΔFosB in the D1-type medium spiny neurons in the nucleus accumbens is necessary and sufficient for many of the neural adaptations and behavioral effects (e.g., expression-dependent increases in drug self-administration and reward sensitization) seen in drug addiction. Once ΔFosB is sufficiently overexpressed, it induces an addictive state that becomes increasingly more severe with further increases in ΔFosB expression. It has been implicated in addictions to alcohol, cannabinoids, cocaine, methylphenidate, nicotine, opioids, phencyclidine, propofol, and substituted amphetamines, among others.

ΔJunD, a transcription factor, and G9a, a histone methyltransferase enzyme, both oppose the function of ΔFosB and inhibit increases in its expression. Sufficiently overexpressing ΔJunD in the nucleus accumbens with viral vectors can completely block many of the neural and behavioral alterations seen in chronic drug abuse (i.e., the alterations mediated by ΔFosB). ΔFosB also plays an important role in regulating behavioral responses to natural rewards, such as palatable food, sex, and exercise. Since both natural rewards and addictive drugs induce expression of ΔFosB (i.e., they cause the brain to produce more of it), chronic acquisition of these rewards can result in a similar pathological state of addiction. Consequently, ΔFosB is the most significant factor involved in both amphetamine addiction and amphetamine-induced sex addictions, which are compulsive sexual behaviors that result from excessive sexual activity and amphetamine use. These sex addictions are associated with a dopamine dysregulation syndrome which occurs in some patients taking dopaminergic drugs.

The effects of amphetamine on gene regulation are both dose- and route-dependent. Most of the research on gene regulation and addiction is based upon animal studies with intravenous amphetamine administration at very high doses. The few studies that have used equivalent (weight-adjusted) human therapeutic doses and oral administration show that these changes, if they occur, are relatively minor. This suggests that medical use of amphetamine does not significantly affect gene regulation.

Pharmacological Treatments

As of May 2014, there is no effective pharmacotherapy for amphetamine addiction. Reviews from 2015 and 2016 indicated that TAAR1-selective agonists have significant therapeutic potential as a treatment for psychostimulant addictions; however, as of February 2016, the only compounds which are known to function as TAAR1-selective agonists are experimental drugs. Amphetamine addiction is largely mediated through increased activation of dopamine receptors and co-localized NMDA receptors in the nucleus accumbens; magnesium ions inhibit NMDA receptors by blocking the receptor calcium channel. One review suggested that, based upon animal testing, pathological (addiction-inducing) psychostimulant use significantly reduces the level of intracellular magnesium throughout the brain. Supplemental magnesium treatment has been shown to reduce amphetamine self-administration (i.e., doses given to oneself) in humans, but it is not an effective monotherapy for amphetamine addiction.

Behavioral Treatments

Cognitive behavioral therapy is currently the most effective clinical treatment for psychostimulant addictions. Additionally, research on the neurobiological effects of physical exercise suggests that daily aerobic exercise, especially endurance exercise (e.g., marathon running), prevents the development of drug addiction and is an effective adjunct therapy (i.e., a supplemental treatment) for amphetamine addiction. Exercise leads to better treatment outcomes when used as an adjunct treatment, particularly for psychostimulant addictions. In particular, aerobic exercise decreases psychostimulant self-administration, reduces the reinstatement (i.e., relapse) of drug-seeking, and induces increased dopamine receptor D_2 (DRD2) density in the striatum. This is the opposite of pathological stimulant use, which induces decreased striatal DRD2 density. One review noted that exercise may also prevent the development of a drug addiction by altering ΔFosB or c-Fos immunoreactivity in the striatum or other parts of the reward system.

Dependence and Withdrawal

According to another Cochrane Collaboration review on withdrawal in individuals who compulsively use amphetamine and methamphetamine, "when chronic heavy users abruptly discontinue amphetamine use, many report a time-limited withdrawal syndrome that occurs within 24 hours of their last dose." This review noted that withdrawal symptoms in chronic, high-dose users are frequent, occurring in up to 87.6% of cases, and persist for three to four weeks with a marked "crash" phase occurring during the first week. Amphetamine withdrawal symptoms can include anxiety, drug craving, depressed mood, fatigue, increased appetite, increased movement or decreased movement, lack of motivation, sleeplessness or sleepiness, and lucid dreams. The review indicated that the severity of withdrawal symptoms is positively correlated with the age of the individual and the extent of their dependence. Manufacturer prescribing information does not indicate the presence of withdrawal symptoms following discontinuation of amphetamine use after an extended period at therapeutic doses.

Toxicity

In rodents and primates, sufficiently high doses of amphetamine cause dopaminergic neurotoxicity, or damage to dopamine neurons, which is characterized by dopamine terminal degeneration and reduced transporter and receptor function. There is no evidence that amphetamine is directly neurotoxic in humans. However, large doses of amphetamine may indirectly cause dopaminergic neurotoxicity as a result of hyperpyrexia, the excessive formation of reactive oxygen species, and increased autoxidation of dopamine. Animal models of neurotoxicity from high-dose amphetamine exposure indicate that the occurrence of hyperpyrexia (i.e., core body temperature ≥ 40° C) is necessary for the development of amphetamine-induced neurotoxicity. Prolonged elevations of brain temperature above 40° C likely promote the development of amphetamine-induced neurotoxicity in laboratory animals by facilitating the production of reactive oxygen species, disrupting cellular protein function, and transiently increasing blood–brain barrier permeability.

Psychosis

A severe amphetamine overdose can result in a stimulant psychosis that may involve a variety of symptoms, such as delusions and paranoia. A Cochrane Collaboration review on treatment for amphetamine, dextroamphetamine, and methamphetamine psychosis states that about 5–15% of users fail to recover completely. According to the same review, there is at least one trial that shows antipsychotic medications effectively resolve the symptoms of acute amphetamine psychosis. Psychosis very rarely arises from therapeutic use.

Interactions

Many types of substances are known to interact with amphetamine, resulting in altered drug action or metabolism of amphetamine, the interacting substance, or both. Inhibitors of the enzymes that metabolize amphetamine (e.g., CYP2D6 and FMO3) will prolong its elimination half-life, meaning that its effects will last longer. Amphetamine also interacts with MAOIs, particularly monoamine oxidase A inhibitors, since both MAOIs and amphetamine increase plasma catecholamines (i.e., norepinephrine and dopamine); therefore, concurrent use of both is dangerous. Amphetamine modulates the activity of most psychoactive drugs. In particular, amphetamine may decrease the effects of sedatives and depressants and increase the effects of stimulants and antidepressants. Amphetamine may also decrease the effects of antihypertensives and antipsychotics due to its effects on blood pressure and dopamine respectively. Zinc supplementation may reduce the minimum effective dose of amphetamine when it is used for the treatment of ADHD.

In general, there is no significant interaction when consuming amphetamine with food, but the pH of gastrointestinal content and urine affects the absorption and excretion of amphetamine, respectively. Acidic substances reduce the absorption of amphetamine and increase urinary excretion, and alkaline substances do the opposite. Due to the effect pH has on absorption, amphetamine also interacts with gastric acid reducers such as proton pump inhibitors and H_2 antihistamines, which increase gastrointestinal pH (i.e., make it less acidic).

Pharmacodynamics

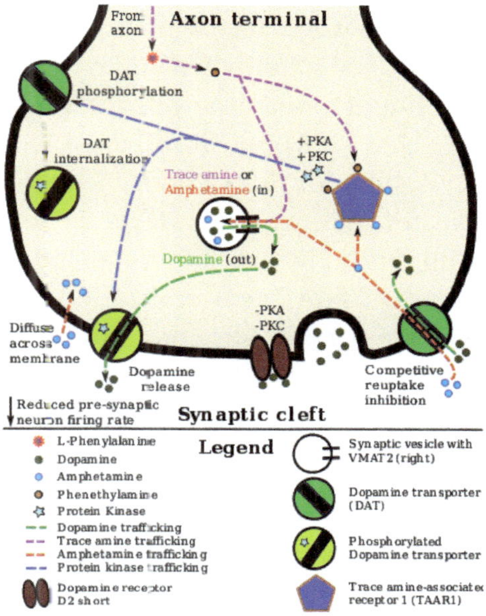

Pharmacodynamics of amphetamine in a dopamine neuron

Amphetamine enters the presynaptic neuron across the neuronal membrane or through DAT. Once inside, it binds to TAAR1 or enters synaptic vesicles through VMAT2. When amphetamine enters synaptic vesicles through VMAT2, it collapses the vesicular pH gradient, which in turn causes dopamine to be released into the cytosol (light tan-colored area) through VMAT2. When amphetamine binds to TAAR1, it reduces the firing rate of the dopamine neuron via potassium channels and activates protein kinase A (PKA) and protein kinase C (PKC), which subsequently phosphorylate DAT. PKA-phosphorylation causes DAT to withdraw into the presynaptic neuron (internalize) and cease transport. PKC-phosphorylated DAT may either operate in reverse or, like PKA-phosphorylated DAT, internalize and cease transport. Amphetamine is also known to increase intracellular calcium, an effect which is associated with DAT phosphorylation through a CAMKIIα-dependent pathway, in turn producing dopamine efflux.

Amphetamine exerts its behavioral effects by altering the use of monoamines as neuronal signals in the brain, primarily in catecholamine neurons in the reward and executive function pathways of the brain. The concentrations of the main neurotransmitters involved in reward circuitry and executive functioning, dopamine and norepinephrine, increase dramatically in a dose-dependent manner by amphetamine due to its effects on monoamine transporters. The reinforcing and motivational salience-promoting effects of amphetamine are mostly due to enhanced dopaminergic activity in the mesolimbic pathway. The euphoric and locomotor-stimulating effects of amphetamine are dependent upon the magnitude and speed by which it increases synaptic dopamine and norepinephrine concentrations in the striatum.

Amphetamine has been identified as a potent full agonist of trace amine-associated receptor 1 (TAAR1), a G_s-coupled and G_q-coupled G protein-coupled receptor (GPCR) discovered in 2001, which is important for regulation of brain monoamines. Activation of TAAR1 increases cAMP production via adenylyl cyclase activation and inhibits monoamine transporter function. Monoamine autoreceptors (e.g., D_2 short, presynaptic α_2, and presynaptic 5-HT_{1A}) have the opposite effect of TAAR1, and together these receptors provide a regulatory system for monoamines. Notably, amphetamine and trace amines bind to TAAR1, but not monoamine autoreceptors. Imaging studies indicate that monoamine reuptake inhibition by amphetamine and trace amines is site specific and depends upon the presence of TAAR1 co-localization in the associated monoamine neurons. As of 2010, co-localization of TAAR1 and the dopamine transporter (DAT) has been visualized in rhesus monkeys, but co-localization of TAAR1 with the norepinephrine transporter (NET) and the serotonin transporter (SERT) has only been evidenced by messenger RNA (mRNA) expression.

In addition to the neuronal monoamine transporters, amphetamine also inhibits both vesicular monoamine transporters, VMAT1 and VMAT2, as well as SLC1A1, SLC22A3, and SLC22A5. SLC1A1 is excitatory amino acid transporter 3 (EAAT3), a glutamate transporter located in neurons, SLC22A3 is an extraneuronal monoamine transporter that is present in astrocytes, and SLC22A5 is a high-affinity carnitine transporter. Amphetamine is known to strongly induce cocaine- and amphetamine-regulated transcript (CART) gene expression, a neuropeptide involved in feeding behavior, stress, and reward, which induces observable increases in neuronal development and survival *in vitro*. The CART receptor has yet to be identified, but there is significant evidence that CART binds to a unique G_i/G_o-coupled GPCR. Amphetamine also inhibits monoamine oxidase at very high doses, resulting in less dopamine and phenethylamine metabolism and consequently higher concentrations of synaptic monoamines. In humans, the only post-synaptic receptor at which amphetamine is known to bind is the 5-HT1A receptor, where it acts as an agonist with micromolar affinity.

The full profile of amphetamine's short-term drug effects in humans is mostly derived through increased cellular communication or neurotransmission of dopamine, serotonin, norepinephrine, epinephrine, histamine, CART peptides, endogenous opioids, adrenocorticotropic hormone, corticosteroids, and glutamate, which it effects through interactions with CART, 5-HT1A, EAAT3, TAAR1, VMAT1, VMAT2, and possibly other biological targets.

Dextroamphetamine is a more potent agonist of TAAR1 than levoamphetamine. Consequently, dextroamphetamine produces greater CNS stimulation than levoamphetamine, roughly three to four times more, but levoamphetamine has slightly stronger cardiovascular and peripheral effects.

Dopamine

In certain brain regions, amphetamine increases the concentration of dopamine in the synaptic cleft. Amphetamine can enter the presynaptic neuron either through DAT or by diffusing across the neuronal membrane directly. As a consequence of DAT uptake, amphetamine produces competitive reuptake inhibition at the transporter. Upon entering the presynaptic neuron, amphetamine activates TAAR1 which, through protein kinase A (PKA) and protein kinase C (PKC) signaling, causes DAT phosphorylation. Phosphorylation by either protein kinase can result in DAT internalization (non-competitive reuptake inhibition), but PKC-mediated phosphorylation alone induces the reversal of dopamine transport through DAT (i.e., dopamine efflux). Amphetamine is also known to increase intracellular calcium, an effect which is associated with DAT phosphorylation through an unidentified Ca2+/calmodulin-dependent protein kinase (CAMK)-dependent pathway, in turn producing dopamine efflux. Through direct activation of G protein-coupled inwardly-rectifying potassium channels, TAAR1 reduces the firing rate of dopamine neurons, preventing a hyper-dopaminergic state.

Amphetamine is also a substrate for the presynaptic vesicular monoamine transporter, VMAT2. Following amphetamine uptake at VMAT2, amphetamine induces the collapse of the vesicular pH gradient, which results in the release of dopamine molecules from synaptic vesicles into the cytosol via dopamine efflux through VMAT2. Subsequently, the cytosolic dopamine molecules are released from the presynaptic neuron into the synaptic cleft via reverse transport at DAT.

Norepinephrine

Similar to dopamine, amphetamine dose-dependently increases the level of synaptic norepinephrine, the direct precursor of epinephrine. Based upon neuronal TAAR1 mRNA expression, amphetamine is thought to affect norepinephrine analogously to dopamine. In other words, amphetamine induces TAAR1-mediated efflux and non-competitive reuptake inhibition at phosphorylated NET, competitive NET reuptake inhibition, and norepinephrine release from VMAT2.

Serotonin

Amphetamine exerts analogous, yet less pronounced, effects on serotonin as on dopamine and norepinephrine. Amphetamine affects serotonin via VMAT2 and, like norepinephrine, is thought to phosphorylate SERT via TAAR1. Like dopamine, amphetamine has low, micromolar affinity at the human 5-HT1A receptor.

Other Neurotransmitters, Peptides, and Hormones

Acute amphetamine administration in humans increases endogenous opioid release in several brain structures in the reward system. Extracellular levels of glutamate, the primary excitatory neurotransmitter in the brain, have been shown to increase in the striatum following exposure to amphetamine. This increase in extracellular glutamate presumably occurs via the amphetamine-induced internalization of EAAT3, a glutamate reuptake transporter, in dopamine neurons. Amphetamine also induces the selective release of histamine from mast cells and efflux from histaminergic neurons through VMAT2. Acute amphetamine administration can also increase adrenocorticotropic hormone and corticosteroid levels in blood plasma by stimulating the hypothalamic–pituitary–adrenal axis.

Pharmacokinetics

The oral bioavailability of amphetamine varies with gastrointestinal pH; it is well absorbed from the gut, and bioavailability is typically over 75% for dextroamphetamine. Amphetamine is a weak base with a pK_a of 9.9; consequently, when the pH is basic, more of the drug is in its lipid soluble free base form, and more is absorbed through the lipid-rich cell membranes of the gut epithelium. Conversely, an acidic pH means the drug is predominantly in a water-soluble cationic (salt) form, and less is absorbed. Approximately 15–40% of amphetamine circulating in the bloodstream is bound to plasma proteins.

The half-life of amphetamine enantiomers differ and vary with urine pH. At normal urine pH, the half-lives of dextroamphetamine and levoamphetamine are 9–11 hours and 11–14 hours, respectively. An acidic diet will reduce the enantiomer half-lives to 8–11 hours; an alkaline diet will increase the range to 16–31 hours. The biological half-life is longer and distribution volumes are larger in amphetamine dependent individuals. The immediate-release and extended release variants of salts of both isomers reach peak plasma concentrations at 3 hours and 7 hours post-dose respectively. Amphetamine is eliminated via the kidneys, with 30–40% of the drug being excreted unchanged at normal urinary pH. When the urinary pH is basic, amphetamine is in its free base form, so less is excreted. When urine pH is abnormal, the urinary recovery of amphetamine may range from a low of 1% to a high of 75%, depending mostly upon whether urine is too basic or acidic, respectively. Amphetamine is usually eliminated within two days of the last oral dose.

The prodrug lisdexamfetamine is not as sensitive to pH as amphetamine when being absorbed in the gastrointestinal tract; following absorption into the blood stream, it is converted by red blood cell-associated enzymes to dextroamphetamine via hydrolysis. The elimination half-life of lisdexamfetamine is generally less than one hour.

CYP2D6, dopamine β-hydroxylase (DBH), flavin-containing monooxygenase 3 (FMO3), butyrate-CoA ligase (XM-ligase), and glycine N-acyltransferase (GLYAT) are the enzymes known to metabolize amphetamine or its metabolites in humans.Amphetamine has a variety of excreted metabolic products, including 4-hydroxyamphetamine, 4-hydroxynorephedrine, 4-hydroxyphenylacetone, benzoic acid, hippuric acid, norephedrine, and phenylacetone. Among these metabolites, the active sympathomimetics are 4hydroxyamphetamine, 4hydroxynorephedrine, and norephedrine. The main metabolic pathways involve aromatic para-hydroxylation, aliphatic alpha- and beta-hydroxylation, N-oxidation, N-dealkylation, and deamination. The known metabolic pathways, detectable metabolites, and metabolizing enzymes in humans include the following:

Metabolic Pathways of Amphetamine in Humans

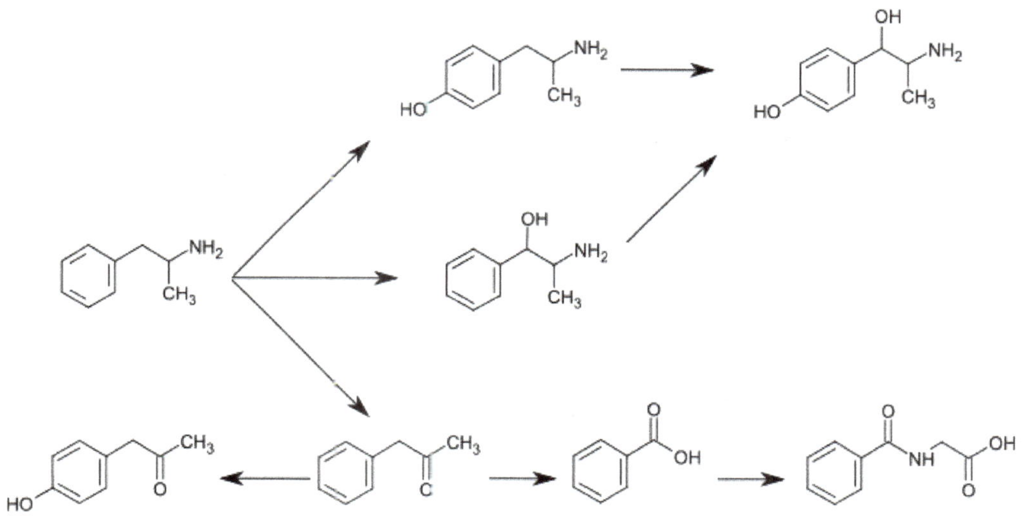

The primary active metabolites of amphetamine are 4-hydroxyamphetamine and norephedrine; at normal urine pH, about 30–40% of amphetamine is excreted unchanged and roughly 50% is excreted as the inactive metabolites (bottom row). The remaining 10–20% is excreted as the active metabolites. Benzoic acid is metabolized by XM-ligase into an intermediate product, benzoyl-CoA, which is then metabolized by GLYAT into hippuric acid.

Related Endogenous Compounds

Amphetamine has a very similar structure and function to the endogenous trace amines, which are naturally occurring neurotransmitter molecules produced in the human body and brain. Among this group, the most closely related compounds are phenethylamine, the parent compound of amphetamine, and *N*-methylphenethylamine, an isomer of amphetamine (i.e., it has an identical molecular formula). In humans, phenethylamine is produced directly from L-phenylalanine by the aromatic amino acid decarboxylase (AADC) enzyme, which converts L-DOPA into dopamine as well. In turn, *N*methylphenethylamine is metabolized from phenethylamine by phenylethanolamine N-methyltransferase, the same enzyme that metabolizes norepinephrine into epinephrine. Like amphetamine, both phenethylamine and *N*methylphenethylamine regulate monoamine neurotransmission via TAAR1; unlike amphetamine, both of these substances are broken down by monoamine oxidase B, and therefore have a shorter half-life than amphetamine.

Chemistry

Racemic Amphetamine

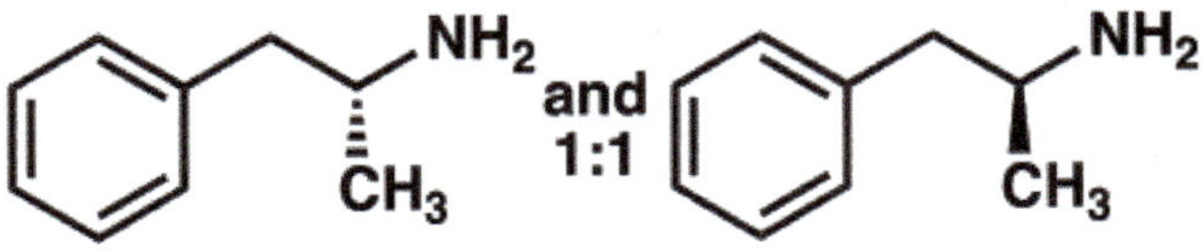

Levoamphetamine Dextroamphetamine

The skeletal structures of L-amph and D-amph

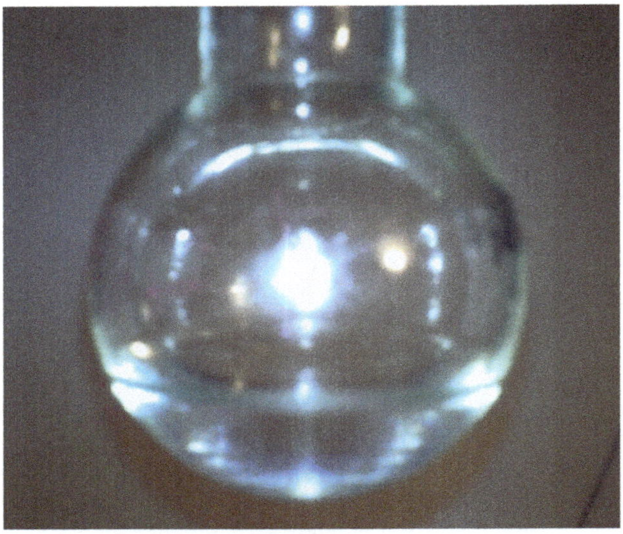

A vial of the colorless amphetamine free base

Amphetamine is a methyl homolog of the mammalian neurotransmitter phenethylamine with the chemical formula $C_9H_{13}N$. The carbon atom adjacent to the primary amine is a stereogenic center, and amphetamine is composed of a racemic 1:1 mixture of two enantiomeric mirror images. This racemic mixture can be separated into its optical isomers: levoamphetamine and dextroamphetamine. At room temperature, the pure free base of amphetamine is a mobile, colorless, and volatile liquid with a characteristically strong amine odor, and acrid, burning taste. Frequently prepared solid salts of amphetamine include amphetamine aspartate, hydrochloride, phosphate, saccharate, and sulfate, the last of which is the most common amphetamine salt. Amphetamine is also the parent compound of its own structural class, which includes a number of psychoactive derivatives. In organic chemistry, amphetamine is an excellent chiral ligand for the stereoselective synthesis of 1,1'-bi-2-naphthol.

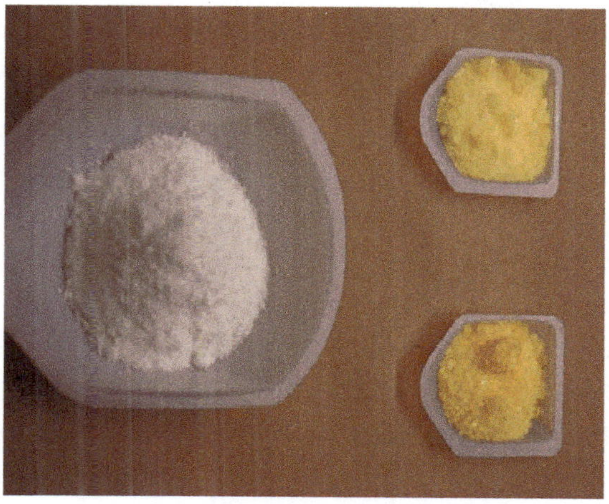

Amphetamine hydrochloride (left bowl)
Phenyl-2-nitropropene (right cups)

Substituted Derivatives

The substituted derivatives of amphetamine, or "substituted amphetamines", are a broad range of chemicals that contain amphetamine as a "backbone"; specifically, this chemical class includes derivative compounds that are formed by replacing one or more hydrogen atoms in the amphetamine core structure with substituents. The class includes amphetamine itself, stimulants like methamphetamine, serotonergic empathogens like MDMA, and decongestants like ephedrine, among other subgroups.

Synthesis

Since the first preparation was reported in 1887, numerous synthetic routes to amphetamine have been developed. The most common route of both legal and illicit amphetamine synthesis employs a non-metal reduction known as the Leuckart reaction (method 1). In the first step, a reaction between phenylacetone and formamide, either using additional formic acid or formamide itself as a reducing agent, yields *N*-formylamphetamine. This intermediate is then hydrolyzed using hydrochloric acid, and subsequently basified, extracted with organic solvent, concentrated, and distilled to yield the free base. The free base is then dissolved in an organic solvent, sulfuric acid added, and amphetamine precipitates out as the sulfate salt.

A number of chiral resolutions have been developed to separate the two enantiomers of amphetamine. For example, racemic amphetamine can be treated with d-tartaric acid to form a diastereoisomeric salt which is fractionally crystallized to yield dextroamphetamine. Chiral resolution remains the most economical method for obtaining optically pure amphetamine on a large scale. In addition, several enantioselective syntheses of amphetamine have been developed. In one example, optically pure (*R*)-1-phenyl-ethanamine is condensed with phenylacetone to yield a chiral Schiff base. In the key step, this intermediate is reduced by catalytic hydrogenation with a transfer of chirality to the carbon atom alpha to the amino group. Cleavage of the benzylic amine bond by hydrogenation yields optically pure dextroamphetamine.

A large number of alternative synthetic routes to amphetamine have been developed based on classic organic reactions. One example is the Friedel–Crafts alkylation of benzene by allyl chloride to yield beta chloropropylbenzene which is then reacted with ammonia to produce racemic amphetamine (method 2). Another example employs the Ritter reaction (method 3). In this route, allylbenzene is reacted acetonitrile in sulfuric acid to yield an organosulfate which in turn is treated with sodium hydroxide to give amphetamine via an acetamide intermediate. A third route starts with ethyl 3-oxobutanoate which through a double alkylation with methyl iodide followed by benzyl chloride can be converted into 2-methyl-3-phenyl-propanoic acid. This synthetic intermediate can be transformed into amphetamine using either a Hofmann or Curtius rearrangement (method 4).

A significant number of amphetamine syntheses feature a reduction of a nitro, imine, oxime or other nitrogen-containing functional groups. In one such example, a Knoevenagel condensation of benzaldehyde with nitroethane yields phenyl-2-nitropropene. The double bond and nitro group of this intermediate is reduced using either catalytic hydrogenation or by treatment with lithium aluminium hydride (method 5). Another method is the reaction of phenylacetone with ammonia, producing an imine intermediate that is reduced to the primary amine using hydrogen over a palladium catalyst or lithium aluminum hydride (method 6).

Detection in Body Fluids

Amphetamine is frequently measured in urine or blood as part of a drug test for sports, employment, poisoning diagnostics, and forensics. Techniques such as immunoassay, which is the most common form of amphetamine test, may cross-react with a number of sympathomimetic drugs. Chromatographic methods specific for amphetamine are employed to prevent false positive results. Chiral separation techniques may be employed to help distinguish the source of the drug, whether prescription amphetamine, prescription amphetamine prodrugs, (e.g., selegiline), over-the-counter drug products that contain levomethamphetamine, or illicitly obtained substituted amphetamines. Several prescription drugs produce amphetamine as a metabolite, including benzphetamine, clobenzorex, famprofazone, fenproporex, lisdexamfetamine, mesocarb, methamphetamine, prenylamine, and selegiline, among others. These compounds may produce positive results for amphetamine on drug tests. Amphetamine is generally only detectable by a standard drug test for approximately 24 hours, although a high dose may be detectable for two to four days.

For the assays, a study noted that an enzyme multiplied immunoassay technique (EMIT) assay for amphetamine and methamphetamine may produce more false positives than liquid chromatography–tandem mass spectrometry. Gas chromatography–mass spectrometry (GC–MS) of amphetamine and methamphetamine with the derivatizing agent

(*S*)-(−)-trifluoroacetylprolyl chloride allows for the detection of methamphetamine in urine. GC–MS of amphetamine and methamphetamine with the chiral derivatizing agent Mosher's acid chloride allows for the detection of both dextroamphetamine and dextromethamphetamine in urine. Hence, the latter method may be used on samples that test positive using other methods to help distinguish between the various sources of the drug.

History, Society, and Culture

Global Estimates of Illegal Drug users in 2014 (In Millions of Users)			
Substance	**Best estimate**	**Low estimate**	**High estimate**
Amphetamine-type stimulants	35.65	15.34	55.90
Cannabis	182.50	127.54	233.65
Cocaine	18.26	14.88	22.08
Ecstasy	19.40	9.89	29.01
Opiates	17.44	13.74	21.59
Opioids	33.12	28.57	38.52

Amphetamine was first synthesized in 1887 in Germany by Romanian chemist Lazăr Edeleanu who named it *phenylisopropylamine*; its stimulant effects remained unknown until 1927, when it was independently resynthesized by Gordon Alles and reported to have sympathomimetic properties. Amphetamine had no pharmacological use until 1934, when Smith, Kline and French began selling it as an inhaler under the trade name Benzedrine as a decongestant. Benzedrine sulfate was introduced three years later and found a wide variety of medical applications, including narcolepsy. During World War II, amphetamine and methamphetamine were used extensively by both the Allied and Axis forces for their stimulant and performance-enhancing effects. As the addictive properties of the drug became known, governments began to place strict controls on the sale of amphetamine. For example, during the early 1970s in the United States, amphetamine became a schedule II controlled substance under the Controlled Substances Act. In spite of strict government controls, amphetamine has been used legally or illicitly by people from a variety of backgrounds, including authors, musicians, mathematicians, and athletes.

Amphetamine is still illegally synthesized today in clandestine labs and sold on the black market, primarily in European countries. Among European Union (EU) member states, 1.2 million young adults used illicit amphetamine or methamphetamine in 2013. During 2012, approximately 5.9 metric tons of illicit amphetamine were seized within EU member states; the "street price" of illicit amphetamine within the EU ranged from €6–38 per gram during the same period. Outside Europe, the illicit market for amphetamine is much smaller than the market for methamphetamine and MDMA.

Legal Status

As a result of the United Nations 1971 Convention on Psychotropic Substances, amphetamine became a schedule II controlled substance, as defined in the treaty, in all (183) state parties. Consequently, it is heavily regulated in most countries. Some countries, such as South Korea and Japan, have banned substituted amphetamines even for medical use. In other nations, such as Canada (schedule I drug), the Netherlands (List I drug), the United States (schedule II drug), Australia (schedule 8), Thailand (category 1 narcotic), and United Kingdom (class B drug), amphetamine is in a restrictive national drug schedule that allows for its use as a medical treatment.

Pharmaceutical Products

Several currently prescribed amphetamine formulations contain both enantiomers, including Adderall, Dyanavel XR, and Evekeo, the last of which is racemic amphetamine sulfate. Amphetamine is also prescribed in enantiopure and prodrug form as dextroamphetamine and lisdexamfetamine respectively. Lisdexamfetamine is structurally different from amphetamine, and is inactive until it metabolizes into dextroamphetamine. The free base of racemic amphetamine was previously available as Benzedrine, Psychedrine, and Sympatedrine. Levoamphetamine was previously available as Cydril. Many current amphetamine pharmaceuticals are salts due to the comparatively high volatility of the free base. However, oral suspension and orally disintegrating tablet (ODT) dosage forms composed of the free base were introduced in 2015 and 2016.

Food Addiction

A food addiction or eating addiction is a behavioral addiction that is characterized by the compulsive consumption of palatable (e.g., high fat and high sugar) foods – the types of food which markedly activate the reward system in humans and other animals – despite adverse consequences.

Psychological dependence has also been observed with the occurrence of withdrawal symptoms when consumption of these foods stops by replacement with foods low in sugar and fat. Professionals address this by providing behavior therapy.

Sugary and high-fat food have both been shown to increase the expression of ΔFosB, an addiction biomarker, in the D1-type medium spiny neurons of the nucleus accumbens; however, there is very little research on the synaptic plasticity from compulsive food consumption, a phenomenon which is known to be caused by ΔFosB overexpression.

Description

"Food addiction" refers to compulsive overeaters who engage in frequent episodes of uncontrolled eating (binge eating). The term *binge eating* means eating an unhealthy amount of food while feeling that one's sense of control has been lost. People who engage in binge eating may feel frenzied, and consume a considerable amount of calories before stopping. The after effects of bingeing in this way is generally followed by feelings of guilt and depression; for example, some will cancel their plans for the next day because they "feel fat." Binge eating also has implications on physical health, due to excessive intake of fats and sugars, which can cause numerous health problems.

Unlike individuals with bulimia nervosa, compulsive overeaters do not attempt to compensate for their bingeing with purging behaviors, such as fasting, laxative use, or vomiting. When compulsive overeaters overeat through binge eating and experience feelings of guilt after their binges, they can be said to have binge eating disorder (BED).

In addition to binge eating, compulsive overeaters may also engage in grazing behavior, during which they continuously eat throughout the day. These actions result in an excessive overall number of calories consumed, even if the quantities eaten at any one time may be small.

During binges, compulsive overeaters may consume between 5,000 and 15,000 food calories daily (far more than is healthy), resulting in a temporary release from psychological stress through an addictive high not unlike that experienced through drug abuse. Compulsive overeaters tend to show brain changes similar to those of drug addicts, a result of excessive consumption of highly processed foods.

For the compulsive overeater, ingesting trigger foods causes the release of the chemical messengers serotonin and dopamine in the brain. This could be another indicator that neurobiological factors contribute to the addictive process. Conversely, abstaining from addictive food and food eating processes causes withdrawal symptoms for those with eating disorders. The resulting decreased levels of serotonin in the individual may trigger higher levels of depression and anxiety.

Eventually, compulsive overeaters continuously think about food. Food is in the preeminent positions of their minds; when deprived of it, the person may engage in actions similar to those of hard drug addicts, including an uncontrollable search for the substance, and in devious behaviour, such as stealing or lying. The problem of obesity is becoming a worldwide problem. A sugar tax is set to be introduced in Ireland to minimise the consumption of harmful foods and drinks.

Signs and Symptoms

A food addiction features compulsive overeating, such as binge eating behavior, as its core and only defining feature. There are several potential signs that a person may be suffering from compulsive overeating. Common behaviors of compulsive overeaters include eating alone, consuming food quickly, and gaining weight rapidly, and eating to the point of feeling sick to the stomach. Other signs include significantly decreased mobility and the withdrawal from activities due to weight gain. Emotional indicators can include feelings of guilt, a sense of loss of control, depression and mood swings.

Hiding consumption is an emotional indicator of other symptoms that could be a result of having a food addiction. Hiding consumption of food includes eating in secret; late at night while everybody else is asleep, in the car, and hiding certain foods until ready to consume in private. Other signs of hiding consumption are avoiding social interactions to eat the specific foods that are craved. Other emotional indicators are Inner guilt; which includes making up excuses to why the palatable food would be beneficial to consume, and then feeling guilty about it shortly after consuming.

Sense of loss of control is indicated in many ways which includes, going out of the way to obtain specific foods, spending unnecessary amounts of money on foods to satisfy cravings. Difficulty concentrating on things such as a job or career can indicate sense of loss of control by not being to organize thoughts leading to a decrease in efficiency. Other ways to indicate the sense of loss of control, are craving food despite being full. One may set rules to try to eat healthy but the cravings over rule and the rules are failed to be followed. One big indicator of loss of control due to food addiction is even though one knows they have a medical problem caused by the craved foods, they cannot stop consuming the foods, which can be detrimental to their health.

Food addiction has some physical signs and symptoms. Decreased energy; not being able to be as active as in the past, not being able to be as active as others around, also a decrease in efficiency due to the lack of energy. Having trouble sleeping; being tired all the time such as fatigue, oversleeping, or the complete opposite and not being able to sleep such as insomnia. Other physical signs and symptoms are restlessness, irritability, digestive disorders, and headaches.

In extreme cases food addiction can result in some suicidal thoughts.

Potential Negative Effects

A Food addiction, especially long-term, can result in negative consequences to all aspects of a person's life, creating damaging and chronic symptoms.

Physical Consequences

The short-term physical effect associated with dopamine and endogenous opiate release in the brain reward center is low level euphoria, a decrease in both anxiety and emotional pain also known as a "food coma." The long-term physical effects may vary. The health consequences can be severe.

If a food addict has obesity, it can be associated with the following:

- diabetes
- high blood pressure
- high cholesterol and triglycerides
- osteoarthritis in the knees
- hips and back
- fungal infections in skin folds that are hard to clean
- congestive heart failure
- shortness of breath
- coronary artery disease
- death.

Psychological Consequences

The psychological and mental effects can prove intense and plague an individual for years. These include hopelessness, powerlessness, isolation, shame, depression, self-loathing, guilt, suicidal thoughts, suicide attempts, and/or self-injurious behaviors.

Relational Consequences

Food addiction impacts relationships, especially those within the family. This is because the person with the addiction is vastly more involved with food than with people – it becomes their safest, most important and meaningful relationship. Other connections to friends and family take a back seat. This often leads to a deep sense of isolation from others.

Management

Compulsive overeating is treatable with nutritional assistance and medication. Psychotherapy may also be required, but recent research has proven this to be useful only as a complementary resource, with short-term effectiveness in middle to severe cases.

Lisdexamfetamine is an FDA-approved appetite suppressant drug that is indicated for the treatment of binge eating disorder. The antidepressant fluoxetine is a medication that is approved by the Food and Drug Administration (FDA) for the treatment of an eating disorder, specifically bulimia nervosa. This medication has been prescribed off-label for the treatment of binge eating disorder (BED). Off-label medications, such as other selective serotonin reuptake inhibitors (SSRIs), have shown some efficacy, as have several atypical agents, such as mianserin, trazodone and bupropion. Anti-obesity medications have also proven very effective. Studies suggest that anti-obesity drugs, or moderate appetite suppressants, may be key to controlling binge eating.

Many eating disorders are thought to be behavioral patterns that stem from emotional struggles; for the individual to develop lasting improvement and a healthy relationship with food, these affective obstacles need to be resolved. Individuals can overcome compulsive overeating through treatment, which should include talk therapy and medical and nutritional counseling. Such counseling has been recently sanctioned by the American Dental Association in their journal article cover-story for the first time in history in 2012: Given "the continued increase in obesity in the United States and the willingness of dentists to assist in prevention and interventional effort, experts in obesity intervention in conjunction with dental educators should develop models of intervention within the scope of dental practice". Moreover, dental appliances such as conventional jaw wiring and orthodontic wiring for controlling compulsive overeating have been shown to be "efficient ways in terms of weight control in properly selected obese patients and usually no serious complications could be encountered through the treatment course.

As well, several twelve-step programs exist to help members recover from compulsive overeating and food addiction, such as Overeaters Anonymous and others.

Epidemiology

A review on behavioral addictions listed the estimated the lifetime prevalence rate (i.e., the proportion of individuals in the population that developed the disorder during their lifetime) for food addiction in the United States as 2.8%.

Gambling Addiction

Problem gambling (or ludomania, but usually referred to as "gambling addiction" or "compulsive gambling") is an urge to gamble continuously despite harmful negative consequences or a desire to stop. Problem gambling is often defined by whether harm is experienced by the gambler or others, rather than by the gambler's behaviour. Severe problem gambling may be diagnosed as clinical pathological gambling if the gambler meets certain criteria. Pathological gambling is a common disorder that is associated with both social and family costs.

The *DSM-5* has re-classified the condition as an addictive disorder, with sufferers exhibiting many similarities to those who have substance addictions. The term *gambling addiction* has long been used in the recovery movement. Pathological gambling was long considered by the American Psychiatric Association to be an impulse control disorder rather than an addiction. However, data suggest a closer relationship between pathological gambling and substance use disorders than exists between PG and obsessive-compulsive disorder, largely because the behaviors in problem gambling and most primary substance use disorders (*i.e.*, those not resulting from a desire to "self-medicate" for another condition such as depression) seek to activate the brain's reward mechanisms while the behaviors characterizing obsessive-compulsive disorder are prompted by overactive and misplaced signals from the brain's fear mechanisms.

Definition

Research by governments in Australia led to a universal definition for that country which appears to be the only research-based definition not to use diagnostic criteria: "Problem gambling is characterized by many difficulties in limiting money and/or time spent on gambling which leads to adverse consequences for the gambler, others, or for the community." The University of Maryland Medical Center defines pathological gambling as "being unable to resist impulses to gamble, which can lead to severe personal or social consequences".

Most other definitions of problem gambling can usually be simplified to any gambling that causes harm to the gambler or someone else in any way; however, these definitions are usually coupled with descriptions of the type of harm or the use of diagnostic criteria. The *DSM-V* has since reclassified pathological gambling as "gambling disorder" and has listed the disorder under substance-related and addictive disorders rather than impulse-control disorders. This is due to the symptomatology of the disorder resembling an addiction not dissimilar to that of substance-abuse. There are both environmental and genetic factors that can influence on gambler and cause some type of addiction. In order to be diagnosed, an individual must have at least four of the following symptoms in a 12-month period:

- Needs to gamble with increasing amounts of money in order to achieve the desired excitement
- Is restless or irritable when attempting to cut down or stop gambling
- Has made repeated unsuccessful efforts to control, cut back, or stop gambling
- Is often preoccupied with gambling (e.g., having persistent thoughts of reliving past gambling experiences, handicapping or planning the next venture, thinking of ways to get money with which to gamble)
- Often gambles when feeling distressed (e.g., helpless, guilty, anxious, depressed)
- After losing money gambling, often returns another day to get even ("chasing" one's losses)

- Lies to conceal the extent of involvement with gambling
- Has jeopardized or lost a significant relationship, job, education or career opportunity because of gambling
- Relies on others to provide money to relieve desperate financial situations caused by gambling

Mechanism and Biology

According to the Illinois Institute for Addiction Recovery, evidence indicates that pathological gambling is an addiction similar to chemical addiction. It has been observed that some pathological gamblers have lower levels of norepinephrine than normal gamblers. According to a study conducted by Alec Roy, formerly at the National Institute on Alcohol Abuse and Alcoholism, norepinephrine is secreted under stress, arousal, or thrill, so pathological gamblers gamble to make up for their under-dosage.

According to a report from Harvard Medical School's division on addictions, there was an experiment constructed where test subjects were presented with situations where they could win, lose, or break even in a casino-like environment. Subjects' reactions were measured using fMRI, a neuroimaging technique. And according to Hans Breiter, co-director of the Motivation and Emotion Neuroscience Center at Massachusetts General Hospital, "monetary reward in a gambling-like experiment produces brain activation very similar to that observed in a cocaine addict receiving an infusion of cocaine." Studies have compared pathological gamblers to substance addicts, concluding that addicted gamblers display more physical symptoms during withdrawal.

Deficiencies in serotonin might also contribute to compulsive behavior, including a gambling addiction. There are three important points discovered after these antidepressant studies:

1. Antidepressants can reduce pathological gambling in case when there is an effect on serotonergic reuptake inhibitors and 5-HT1/5-HT2 receptor antagonists.
2. Pathological gambling, as the part of obsessive-compulsive disorder, requires the higher doses of antidepressants as it usually required for depressive disorders.
3. In cases where participants do not have or have minimal symptoms of anxiety or depression, antidepressants still have those effect.

A limited study was presented at a conference in Berlin, suggesting opioid release differs in problem gamblers form the general population, but in a very different way from alcoholics or other substance abusers.

The findings in one review indicated the sensitization theory is responsible. Dopamine dysregulation syndrome has been observed in the aforementioned theory in people with regard to such activities as gambling.

Some medical authors suggest that the biomedical model of problem gambling may be unhelpful because it focuses only on individuals. These authors point out that social factors may be a far more important determinant of gambling behaviour than brain chemicals and they suggest that a social model may be more useful in understanding the issue. For example, an apparent increase in problem gambling in the UK may be better understood as a consequence of changes in legislation which came into force in 2007 and enabled casinos, bookmakers, and online betting sites to advertise on TV and radio for the first time and which eased restrictions on the opening of betting shops and online gambling sites.

Relation to Other Problems

Pathological gambling is similar to many other impulse control disorders such as kleptomania. According to evidence from both community- and clinic-based studies, individuals who are pathological gamblers are highly likely to exhibit other psychiatric problems concurrently, including substance use disorders, mood and anxiety disorders, or personality disorders.

Pathological gambling shows several similarities with substance abuse. There is a partial overlap in diagnostic criteria; pathological gamblers are also likely to abuse alcohol and other drugs. The "telescoping phenomenon" reflects the rapid development from initial to problematic behavior in women compared with men. This phenomenon was initially described for alcoholism, but it has also been applied to pathological gambling. Also biological data provide a support for a relationship between pathological gambling and substance abuse.

In a 1995 survey of 184 Gamblers Anonymous members in Illinois, Illinois State professor Henry Lesieur found that 56 percent admitted to some illegal act to obtain money to gamble. Fifty-eight percent admitted they wrote bad checks, while 44 percent said they stole or embezzled money from their employer. Compulsive gambling can affect personal relationships. In a 1991 study of relationships of American men, it was found that 10% of compulsive gamblers had been married more than twice. Only 2% of men who did not gamble were married more than twice. According to statistics by the BGM, families of problem gamblers are more likely to experience child abuse or other forms of domestic violence. According to John A. Cunningham, Joanne Cordingley, David C. Higgins and Tony Toneatto a survey based in Canada shows that gambling abuse was best seen as a form of "disease or illness", "wrongdoing", "habit not disease" and an "addiction similar to drug addiction".

Suicide Rates

A gambler who does not receive treatment for pathological gambling when in his or her desperation phase may contemplate suicide. Problem gambling is often associated with increased suicidal ideation and attempts compared to the general population.

Early onset of problem gambling increases the lifetime risk of suicide. However, gambling-related suicide attempts are usually made by older people with problem gambling. Both comorbid substance use and comorbid mental disorders increase the risk of suicide in people with problem gambling. A 2010 Australian hospital study found that 17% of suicidal patients admitted to the Alfred Hospital's emergency department were problem gamblers. In the United States, a report by the National Council on Problem Gambling showed approximately one in five pathological gamblers attempt suicide. The council also said that suicide rates among pathological gamblers were higher than any other addictive disorder.

David Phillips, a sociologist from the University of California-San Diego, found "visitors to and residents of gaming communities experience significantly elevated suicide levels". According to him, Las Vegas, the largest gaming market in the United States, "displays the highest levels of suicide in the nation, both for residents of Las Vegas and for visitors to that setting". In Atlantic City, the second-largest gaming market, he found "abnormally high suicide levels for visitors and residents appeared only after gambling casinos were opened".

Psychological Mechanisms

Several psychological mechanisms are thought to be implicated in the development and maintenance of problem gambling. First, reward processing seems to be less sensitive with problem gamblers. Second, some individuals use problem gambling as an escape from the problems in their lives (an example of negative reinforcement). Third, personality factors play a role, such as narcissism, risk-seeking, sensation-seeking and impulsivity. Fourth, problem gamblers suffer from a number of cognitive biases, including the illusion of control, unrealistic optimism, overconfidence and the gambler's fallacy (the incorrect belief that a series of random events tends to self-correct so that the absolute frequencies of each of various outcomes balance each other out). Fifth, problem gamblers represent a chronic state of a behavioral spin process, a gambling spin, as described by the criminal spin theory.

Diagnosis

The most common instrument used to screen for "probable pathological gambling" behavior is the South Oaks Gambling Screen (SOGS) developed by Lesieur and Blume (1987) at the South Oaks Hospital in New York City. In recent years the use of SOGS has declined due to a number of criticisms, including that it overestimates false positives (Battersby, Tolchard, Thomas & Esterman, 2002).

The *DSM-IV* diagnostic criteria presented as a checklist is an alternative to SOGS, it focuses on the psychological motivations underpinning problem gambling and was developed by the American Psychiatric Association. It consists of ten diagnostic criteria. One frequently used screening measure based upon the DSM-IV criteria is the National Opinion Research Center DSM Screen for Gambling Problems (NODS). The Canadian Problem Gambling Inventory (CPGI) and the Victorian Gambling Screen (VGS) are newer assessment measures. The Problem Gambling Severity Index, which focuses on the harms associated with problem gambling, is composed of nine items from the longer CPGI. The VGS is also harm based and includes 15 items. The VGS has proven validity and reliability in population studies as well as Adolescents and clinic gamblers.

Treatment

Most treatment for problem gambling involves counseling, step-based programs, self-help, peer-support, medication, or a combination of these. However, no one treatment is considered to be most efficacious and no medications have been approved for the treatment of pathological gambling by the U.S. Food and Drug Administration (FDA). Only one treatment facility has been given a license to officially treat gambling as an addiction, and that was by the State of Virginia.

Gamblers Anonymous (GA) is a commonly used treatment for gambling problems. Modeled after Alcoholics Anonymous, GA uses a 12-step model that emphasizes a mutual-support approach. There are three in-patient treatment centers in North America. One form of counseling, cognitive behavioral therapy (CBT) has been shown to reduce symptoms and gambling-related urges. This type of therapy focuses on the identification of gambling-related thought processes, mood and cognitive distortions that increase one's vulnerability to out-of-control gambling. Additionally, CBT approaches frequently utilize skill-building techniques geared toward relapse prevention, assertiveness and gambling refusal, problem solving and reinforcement of gambling-inconsistent activities and interests.

As to behavioral treatment, some recent research supports the use of both activity scheduling and desensitization in the treatment of gambling problems. In general, behavior analytic research in this area is growing There is evidence that the SSRI paroxetine is efficacious in the treatment of pathological gambling. Additionally, for patients suffering from both pathological gambling and a comorbid bipolar spectrum condition, sustained release lithium has shown efficacy in a preliminary trial. The opioid antagonist drug nalmefene has also been trialled quite successfully for the treatment of compulsive gambling.

Step-based Programs

Other step-based programs are specific to gambling and generic to healing addiction, creating financial health, and improving mental wellness. Commercial alternatives that are designed for clinical intervention, using the best of health science and applied education practices, have been used as patient-centered tools for intervention since 2007. They include measured efficacy and resulting recovery metrics.

Motivational Interviewing

Motivational interviewing is one of the treatments of compulsive gambling. The motivational interviewing's basic goal is promoting readiness to change through thinking and resolving mixed feelings. Avoiding aggressive confrontation, argument, labeling, blaming, and direct persuasion, the interviewer supplies empathy and advice to compulsive gamblers who define their own goal. The focus is on promoting freedom of choice and encouraging confidence in the ability to change.

Peer Support

A growing method of treatment is peer support. With the advancement of online gambling, many gamblers experiencing issues use various online peer-support groups to aid their recovery. This protects their anonymity while allowing them to attempt recovery on their own, often without having to disclose their issues to loved ones.

Self-help

Research into self-help for problem gamblers has shown benefits. A study by Wendy Slutske of the University of Missouri concluded one-third of pathological gamblers overcome it by natural recovery.

Impact (Australia)

According to the Productivity Commission's 2010 final report into gambling, the social cost of problem gambling is close to 4.7 billion dollars a year. Some of the harms resulting from problem gambling include depression, suicide, lower work productivity, job loss, relationship breakdown, crime and bankruptcy. A survey conducted in 2008 found that the most common motivation for fraud was problem gambling, with each incident averaging a loss of $1.1 million. According to Darren R. Christensen. Nicki A. Dowling, Alun C. Jackson and Shane A.Thomas a survey done from 1994-2008 in Tasmania gave results that gambling participation rates have risen rather than fallen over this period.

Prevalence Europe

In Europe, the rate of problem gambling is typically 0.5 to 3 percent. The "British Gambling Prevalence Survey 2007", conducted by the United Kingdom Gambling Commission, found approximately 0.6 percent of the adult population had problem gambling issues—the same percentage as in 1999. The highest prevalence of problem gambling was found among those who participated in spread betting (14.7%), fixed odds betting terminals (11.2%) and betting exchanges (9.8%). In Norway, a December 2007 study showed the amount of present problem gamblers was 0.7 percent.

North America

In the United States, the percentage of pathological gamblers was 0.6 percent, and the percentage of problem gamblers was 2.3 percent in 2008. Studies commissioned by the National Gambling Impact Study Commission Act has shown the prevalence rate ranges from 0.1 percent to 0.6 percent. Nevada has the highest percentage of pathological gambling; a 2002 report estimated 2.2 to 3.6 percent of Nevada residents over the age of 18 could be called problem gamblers. Also, 2.7 to 4.3 percent could be called probable pathological gamblers.

According to a 1997 meta-analysis by Harvard Medical School's division on addictions, 1.1 percent of the adult population of the United States and Canada could be called pathological gamblers. A 1996 study estimated 1.2 to 1.9 percent of adults in Canada were pathological. In Ontario, a 2006 report showed 2.6 percent of residents experienced "moderate gambling problems" and 0.8 percent had "severe gambling problems". In Quebec, an estimated 0.8 percent of the adult population were pathological gamblers in 2002. Although most who gamble do so without harm, approximately 6 million American adults are addicted to gambling.

Signs of a gambling problem include:

- Using income or savings to gamble while letting bills go unpaid
- Repeated, unsuccessful attempts to stop gambling
- Chasing losses
- Losing sleep over thoughts of gambling
- Arguing with friends or family about gambling behavior
- Feeling depressed or suicidal because of gambling losses

Oceania (Australia)

Both casinos and poker machines in pubs and clubs facilitate problem gambling in Australia. The building of new hotels and casinos has been described as "one of the most active construction markets in Australia"; for example, AUD$860 million was allocated to rebuild and expand the Star Complex in Sydney.

A 2010 study, conducted in the Northern Territory by researchers from the Australian National University (ANU) and Southern Cross University (SCU), found that the proximity of a person's residence to a gambling venue is significant in terms of prevalence. Harmful gambling in the study was prevalent among those living within 100 metres of any gambling venue, and was over 50% higher than among those living ten kilometres from a venue. The study's data stated:

"Specifically, people who lived 100 metres from their favourite venue visited an estimated average of 3.4 times per month. This compared to an average of 2.8 times per month for people living one kilometre away, and 2.2 times per month for people living ten kilometres away".

According to the Productivity Commission's 2016 report into gambling, 0.5% to 1% (80,000 to 160,000) of the Australian adult population suffered with significant problems resulting from gambling. A further 1.4% to 2.1% (230 000 to 350 000) of the Australian adult population experienced moderate risks making them likely to be vulnerable to problem gambling. Estimates show that problem gamblers account for an average of 41% of the total gaming machine spending.

Sexual Addiction

Sexual addiction, also known as sex addiction, is a state characterized by compulsive participation or engagement in sexual activity, particularly sexual intercourse, despite negative consequences. Proponents of a diagnostic model for sexual addiction, as defined here, consider it to be one of several sex-related disorders within an umbrella concept known as hypersexual disorder. The term *sexual dependence* is also used to refer to people who report being unable to control their sexual urges, behaviors, or thoughts. Related models of pathological sexual behavior include hypersexuality (nymphomania and satyriasis), erotomania, Don Juanism (or Don Juanitaism), and paraphilia-related disorders.

The concept of sexual addiction is contentious. There is considerable debate amongst psychiatrists, psychologists, sexologists, and other specialists over the whether compulsive sexual behavior constitutes an addiction, and therefore its classification and possible diagnosis. As of 2017, sexual addiction is not a clinical diagnosis in either the DSM or ICD medical classifications of diseases and medical disorders. Some argue that applying such concepts to normal behaviors such as sex, can be problematic, and suggest that applying medical models such as addiction to human sexuality can serve to pathologise normal behavior and cause harm.

Neuroscientists, pharmacologists, molecular biologists, and other researchers in related fields have identified the transcriptional and epigenetic mechanisms of addiction pathophysiology. Diagnostic models, which use the pharmacological model of addiction (this model associates addiction with drug-related concepts, particularly physical dependence, drug withdrawal, and drug tolerance), do not currently include diagnostic criteria to identify sexual addictions in a clinical setting. In the brain disease model of addiction, which uses neuropsychological concepts to characterize addictions, sexual addictions are identifiable and well-characterized. In this model, addictive drugs are characterized as those which are both reinforcing and rewarding. Addictive behaviors (those which can induce a compulsive state) are similarly identified and characterized by their rewarding and reinforcing properties.

Mechanisms

Current neuroscience research on compulsive sexual behavior indicates that it is well-characterized as an addiction and that it develops through the same biomolecular mechanisms that induce drug addictions. Sexual activity is an intrinsic reward that has been shown to act as a positive reinforcer, strongly activate the reward system, and induce the accumulation of ΔFosB in part of the striatum (specifically, the nucleus accumbens). Chronic and excessive activation of certain pathways within the reward system and the accumulation of ΔFosB in a specific group of neurons within the nucleus accumbens has been directly implicated in the development of the compulsive behavior that characterizes addiction.

In humans, a dopamine dysregulation syndrome, characterized by drug-induced compulsive engagement in sexual activity or gambling, has also been observed in some individuals taking dopaminergic medications. Current experimental models of addiction to natural rewards and drug reward demonstrate common alterations in gene expression in the mesocorticolimbic projection. ΔFosB is the most significant gene transcription factor involved in addiction, since its viral or genetic overexpression in the nucleus accumbens is necessary and sufficient for most of the neural adaptations and plasticity that occur; it has been implicated in addictions to alcohol, cannabinoids, cocaine, nicotine, opioids, phenylcyclidine, and substituted amphetamines. ΔJunD is the transcription factor which directly opposes ΔFosB. Increases in nucleus accumbens ΔJunD expression can reduce or, with a large increase, even block most of the neural alterations seen in chronic drug abuse (i.e., the alterations mediated by ΔFosB).

ΔFosB also plays an important role in regulating behavioral responses to natural rewards, such as palatable food, sex, and exercise. Natural rewards, like drugs of abuse, induce ΔFosB in the nucleus accumbens, and chronic acquisition of these rewards can result in a similar pathological addictive state. Thus, ΔFosB is also the key transcription factor involved in addictions to natural rewards as well, and sex addictions in particular, since ΔFosB in the nucleus accumbens is critical for the reinforcing effects of sexual reward. Research on the interaction between natural and drug rewards suggests that psychostimulants and sexual reward possess cross-sensitization effects and act on common biomolecular mechanisms of addiction-related neuroplasticity which are mediated through ΔFosB.

Diagnosis

None of the official diagnostic classification frameworks list "sexual addiction" as a distinct disorder.

DSM

The American Psychiatric Association (APA) publishes and periodically updates the Diagnostic and Statistical Manual of Mental Disorders (DSM), a widely recognized compendium of mental health diagnostics.

The version published in 1987 (DSM-III-R), referred to "distress about a pattern of repeated sexual conquests or other forms of nonparaphilic sexual addiction, involving a succession of people who exist only as things to be used." The reference to sexual addiction was subsequently removed. The DSM-IV-TR, published in 2000 (DSM-IV-TR), did not include sexual addiction as a mental disorder.

Some authors suggested that sexual addiction should be re-introduced into the DSM system; however, sexual addiction was rejected for inclusion in the DSM-5, which was published in 2013. Darrel Regier, vice-chair of the DSM-5 task force, said that "lthough 'hypersexuality' is a proposed new addition...[the phenomenon] was not at the point where we were ready to call it an addiction." The proposed diagnosis does not make the cut as an official diagnosis due to a lack of research into diagnostic criteria for compulsive sexual behavior, according to the APA.

ICD

The World Health Organization produces the International Classification of Diseases (ICD), which is not limited to mental disorders. The most recent version of that document, ICD-10, includes "excessive sexual drive" as a diagnosis (code F52.8), subdividing it into *satyriasis* (for males) and *nymphomania* (for females). However, the ICD categorises these diagnoses as compulsive behaviors or impulse control disorders and not addiction.

CCMD

The Chinese Society of Psychiatry produces the Chinese Classification of Mental Disorders (CCMD), which is currently in its third edition – the CCMD-3 does not include sexual addiction as a diagnosis.

Other Diagnostic Criteria

Some mental health providers have proposed various, but similar, criteria for diagnosing sexual addiction, including Patrick Carnes, and Aviel Goodman. Carnes authored the first clinical book about sex addiction in 1983, based on his own empirical research. His diagnostic model is still largely utilized by the thousands of certified sex addiction therapists (CSATs) trained by the organization he founded. No diagnostic proposal for sex addiction has been adopted into any official government diagnostic manual, however.

During the update of the Diagnostic and Statistical Manual to version 5 (DSM-5), the APA rejected two independent proposals for inclusion.

In 2011, the American Society of Addiction Medicine (ASAM), the largest medical consensus of physicians dedicated to treating and preventing addiction, redefined addiction as a chronic brain disorder, which for the first time broadened the definition of addiction from substances to include addictive behaviors and reward-seeking, such as gambling and sex.

Borderline Personality Disorder

The ICD, DSM and CCMD list promiscuity as a prevalent and problematic symptom for Borderline Personality Disorder. Individuals with this diagnosis sometimes engage in sexual behaviors which can appear out of control causing distress to the individual or attracting negative reception from others. There is therefore a risk that a person presenting with sex addiction, may in fact be suffering from Borderline Personality Disorder. This may lead to inappropriate or incomplete treatment.

Medical Reviews and Position Statements

In November 2016, the American Association of Sexuality Educators, Counselors and Therapists (AASECT), the official body for sex and relationship therapy in the United States, issued a position statement on Sex Addiction which states that AASECT "does not find sufficient empirical evidence to support the classification of sex addiction or porn addiction as a mental health disorder, and does not find the sexual addiction training and treatment methods and educational pedagogies to be adequately informed by accurate human sexuality knowledge. Therefore, it is the position of AASECT that linking problems related to sexual urges, thoughts or behaviors to a porn/sexual addiction process cannot be advanced by AASECT as a standard of practice for sexuality education delivery, counseling or therapy."

Treatment

Psychosexual Therapy / Sex and Relationship Counselling

As of 2017, none of the official regulatory bodies for Psychosexual Counselling or Sex and Relationship therapy, have accepted sex addiction as a distinct entity with associated treatment protocols. Indeed, some practitioners regard sex addiction to be a potentially harmful diagnosis and draw parallels with gay conversion therapy. As a result, treatment for sex addiction is more often provided by addiction professionals than psychosexual specialists.

Addiction Treatment and Recovery Programs

The addiction field has recently set up specialist organisations to provide support to people who feel they may have a sex addiction problem. These include ATSAC (the Association for the Treatment of Sexual Addiction and Compulsivity) in the UK and CSAT (Certified Sex Addiction Therapists) in the US.

Cognitive behavioral therapy is a common form of behavioral treatment for addictions and maladaptive behaviors in general. Dialectical behavior therapy has been shown to improve treatment outcomes as well. Certified Sex Addiction Therapists (CSAT) – a group of sexual addiction therapists certified by the International Institute for Trauma and Addiction Professionals – offer specialized behavioral therapy designed specifically for sexual addiction.

Support Groups

Online Support Groups

NoFap is an online community founded in 2011. It serves as a support group for those who wish to avoid the use of pornography, masturbation, and/or sexual intercourse.

In-person Support Groups

In-person support groups are available in most of the developed world. These groups include:

- Sex Addicts Anonymous: For those who want to reduce or eliminate their use of pornography, masturbation, and/or unwanted sexual activity.
- Sex and Love Addicts Anonymous: Similar to the above.
- Sexaholics Anonymous: For those who want to eliminate their use of pornography, masturbation, unwanted sexual activity, and/or sex outside of marriage. Has a stricter definition of sexual sobriety than its competitors.
- Smart Recovery.

In places where none of the above are available, open meetings of Alcoholics Anonymous or Narcotics Anonymous may be a second-best option.

Support groups may be useful for uninsured or under-insured individuals. They may also be useful as an adjunct to professional treatment. In addition, they may be useful in places where professional practices are full (i.e. not accepting new patients), scarce, or nonexistent, or where these practices have waiting lists. Finally, they may be useful for patients who are reluctant to spend money on professional treatment.

Medications

Behavioral addiction is a treatable condition. Treatment options include psychotherapy and psychopharmacotherapy (i.e., medications) or a combination of both. Cognitive behavioral therapy (CBT) is the most common form of psychotherapy used in treating behavioral addictions; it focuses on identifying patterns that trigger compulsive behavior and making lifestyle changes to promote healthier behaviors. Currently, there are no medications approved for treatment of behavioral addictions in general, but some medications used for treatment of drug addiction may also be beneficial with specific behavioral addictions.

Epidemiology

According to a systematic review from 2014, prevalence rates of sexual addiction and related sexual disorders ranges from 3% to 6%.

History

Sex addiction as a term first emerged in the mid-1970s when various members of Alcoholics Anonymous sought to apply the principles of 12-steps toward sexual recovery from serial infidelity and other unmanageable compulsive sex behaviors that were similar to the powerlessness and un-manageability they experienced with alcoholism. Multiple 12-step style self-help groups now exist for people who identify as sex addicts, including Sex Addicts Anonymous, Sexaholics Anonymous, Sex and Love Addicts Anonymous, and Sexual Compulsives Anonymous.

Society and Culture

Controversy

The controversy surrounding sexual addiction is centered around its identification, through a diagnostic model, in a clinical setting. As noted in current medical literature reviews, compulsive sexual behavior has been observed in humans; drug-induced compulsive sexual behavior has also been noted clinically in some individuals taking dopaminergic drugs. Moreover, current medical research involving neuropsychological models has identified sexual addictions (i.e., the compulsive engagement in sexual behavior despite negative consequences) as a true form of addiction (i.e., it possesses all the necessary characteristics to classify it as one) in animal models. Since current diagnostic models use drug-related concepts as diagnostic criteria for addictions, these are ill-suited for modelling compulsive behaviors in a clinical setting. Consequently, diagnostic classification systems, such as the DSM, do not include sexual addiction as a diagnosis because there is currently "insufficient peer-reviewed evidence to establish the diagnostic criteria and course descriptions needed to identify these behaviors as mental disorders". A 2014 systematic review on sexual addiction indicated that the "lack of empirical evidence on sexual addiction is the result of the disease's complete absence from versions of the Diagnostic and Statistical Manual of Mental Disorders."

There have been debates regarding the definition and existence of sexual addictions for decades, as the issue was covered in a 1994 journal article. According to a 2014 systematic review, sexual addiction (including excessive masturbation and pornography addiction) is a diagnosable behavioral addiction with estimable prevalence rates. The Mayo Clinic considers sexual addiction to be a form of obsessive compulsive disorder and refer to it as *sexual compulsivity* (note that by definition, an addiction is a compulsion toward rewarding stimuli). A paper dating back to 1988 and a journal comment letter published in 2006 asserted that sex addiction is itself a myth, a by-product of cultural and other influences. The 1988 paper argued that the condition is instead a way of projecting social stigma onto patients.

In a non-academic opinion report from 2003, Marty Klein, stated that "the concept of sex addiction provides an excellent example of a model that is both sex-negative and politically disastrous." Klein singled out a number of features that he considered crucial limitations of the sex addiction model and stated that the diagnostic criteria for sexual addiction are easy to find on the internet. Drawing on the *Sexual Addiction Screening Test*, he stated that "the sexual addiction diagnostic criteria make problems of nonproblematic experiences, and as a result pathologize a majority of people."

Popular Culture

Sexual addiction has been the main theme in a variety of films including *Diary of a Sex Addict*, *I Am a Sex Addict*, *Black Snake Moan*, *Confessions of a Porn Addict*, *Shame*, *Thanks for Sharing*, *Choke*, *The Truth* and others.

Behavioral Addiction

Behavioral addiction is a form of addiction that involves a compulsion to engage in a rewarding non-drug-related behavior – sometimes called a natural reward – despite any negative consequences to the person's physical, mental, social or financial well-being. A gene transcription factor known as ΔFosB has been identified as a necessary common factor involved in both behavioral and drug addictions, which are associated with the same set of neural adaptations in the reward system.

Biomolecular Mechanisms

ΔFosB, a gene transcription factor, has been identified as playing a critical role in the development of addictive states in both behavioral addictions and drug addictions. Overexpression of ΔFosB in the nucleus accumbens is necessary and sufficient for many of the neural adaptations seen in drug addiction; it has been implicated in addictions to alcohol, cannabinoids, cocaine, nicotine, phenylcyclidine, and substituted amphetamines as well as addictions to natural rewards such as sex, exercise, and food. A recent study also demonstrated a cross-sensitization between drug reward (amphetamine) and a natural reward (sex) that was mediated by ΔFosB.

Besides increased ΔFosB expression in the nucleus accumbens, there are many other correlations in the neurobiology of behavioral addictions with drug addictions.

One of the most important discoveries of addictions has been the drug based reinforcement and, even more important, reward based learning processes. Several structures of the brain are important in the conditioning process of behavioral addiction; these subcortical structures form the brain regions known as the reward system. One of the major areas of study is the amygdala, a brain structure which involves emotional significance and associated learning. Research shows that dopaminergic projections from the ventral tegmental area facilitate a motivational or learned association to a specific behavior. Dopamine neurons take a role in the learning and sustaining of many acquired behaviors. Research specific to Parkinson's disease has led to identifying the intracellular signaling pathways that underlie the immediate actions of dopamine. The most common mechanism of dopamine is to create addictive properties along with certain behaviors. There are three stages to the dopamine reward system: bursts of dopamine, triggering of behavior, and further impact to the behavior. Once electronically signaled, possibly through the behavior, dopamine neurons let out a 'burst-fire' of elements to stimulate areas along fast transmitting pathways. The behavior response then perpetuates the striated neurons to further send stimuli. The fast firing of dopamine neurons can be monitored over time by evaluating the amount of extracellular concentrations of dopamine through micro dialysis and brain imaging. This monitoring can lead to a model in which one can see the multiplicity of triggering over a period of time. Once the behavior is triggered, it is hard to work away from the dopamine reward system.

Behaviors like gambling have been linked to the new found idea of the brain's capacity to anticipate rewards. The reward system can be triggered by early detectors of the behavior, and trigger dopamine neurons to begin stimulating behaviors. But in some cases, it can lead to many issues due to error, or reward-prediction errors. These errors can act as teaching signals to create a complex behavior task over time.

Psychiatric and Medical Classifications

Diagnostic models do not currently include the criteria necessary to identify behaviors as addictions in a clinical setting. Behavioral addictions has been proposed as a new class in DSM-5, but the only category included is gambling addiction. Internet gaming addiction is included in the appendix as a condition for further study.

Behavioral addictions, which are sometimes referred to as impulse control disorders, are increasingly recognized as treatable forms of addiction. The type of excessive behaviors identified as being addictive include gambling, food, sexual intercourse, use of pornography, use of computers, playing video games, use of the internet, exercise, and shopping.

Researching addiction to food, for example, a 2009 Scripps Research Institute study found evidence that the same molecular mechanisms correlated with human drug addiction also exist in compulsive overeating in obese rats. The dopamine D_2 receptor studied is associated with vulnerability to drug addiction in humans. It was found downregulated in obese rats exposed to a high fat diet, and further reductions of the receptor increased compulsive eating. The D_2 receptor responds to dopamine, a central neurotransmitter released in anticipation of rewarding, satiating experiences such as those involving food, sex or psychoactive drugs.

On August 15, 2011 the American Society of Addiction Medicine (ASAM) issued a public statement defining all addiction in terms of brain changes. "Addiction is a primary, chronic disease of brain reward, motivation, memory and related circuitry."

The following excerpts are taken from the organization's FAQs:

The new ASAM definition makes a departure from equating addiction with just substance dependence, by describing how addiction is also related to behaviors that are rewarding. This is the first time that ASAM has taken an official position that addiction is not solely "substance dependence." This definition says that addiction is about functioning and brain circuitry and how the structure and function of the brains of persons with addiction differ from the structure and function of the brains of persons who do not have addiction. It talks about reward circuitry in the brain and related circuitry, but the emphasis is not on the external rewards that act on the reward system. Food and sexual behaviors and gambling behaviors can be associated with the "pathological pursuit of rewards" described in this new definition of addiction.

We all have the brain reward circuitry that makes food and sex rewarding. In fact, this is a survival mechanism. In a healthy brain, these rewards have feedback mechanisms for satiety or 'enough.' In someone with addiction, the circuitry becomes dysfunctional such that the message to the individual becomes 'more', which leads to the pathological pursuit of rewards and/or relief through the use of substances and behaviors. So, anyone who has addiction is vulnerable to food and sex addiction.

Since ASAM released its statement, and shortly before its release, additional new studies have come out on Internet addiction. They reveal the same fundamental brain changes seen in other addicts of drugs. Another 2011 study found that the risk of Internet addiction in men was about three times more than women. Researchers noted:

> Internet addiction is a psychosocial disorder and its characteristics are as follows: tolerance, withdrawal symptoms, affective disorders, and problems in social relations. Internet usage creates psychological, social, school and/or work difficulties in a person's life. Eighteen percent of study participants were considered to be pathological Internet users, whose excessive use of the Internet was causing academic, social, and interpersonal problems. Excessive Internet use may create a heightened level of psychological arousal, resulting in little sleep,

failure to eat for long periods, and limited physical activity, possibly leading to the user experiencing physical and mental health problems such as depression, OCD, low family relationships and anxiety.

Treatment

Behavioral addiction is a treatable condition. Treatment options include psychotherapy and psychopharmacotherapy (i.e., medications) or a combination of both. Cognitive behavioral therapy (CBT) is the most common form of psychotherapy used in treating behavioral addictions; it focuses on identifying patterns that trigger compulsive behavior and making lifestyle changes to promote healthier behaviors. Currently, there are no medications approved for treatment of behavioral addictions in general, but some medications used for treatment of drug addiction may also be beneficial with specific behavioral addictions. Any unrelated psychiatric disorders should be kept under control, and differentiated from the contributing factors that cause the addiction.

Shopping Addiction

Shopping addiction is defined as the deficiency of impulse control which appears as the eagerness for constantly making new purchases of unnecessary or superfluous things. It is a concept similar to "compulsive buying disorder" and "oniomania", although these terms usually have a more clinical approach, related to a psychological individual disorder of impulse control. The phrase "shopping addiction" usually has a more psychosocial perspective . or it is placed among drug-free addictions like the addiction to gambling, Internet, or video-games.

Behavioural Manifestations

There are three kinds of behavioural manifestations of shopping addiction, with different repercussions. These can be displayed together or independently and in more or less intense ways. Nevertheless, they are closely related and appear joined in people who seriously suffer from this disorder.

First is the attraction towards the consumer stimulus, which is the addiction to purchasing as a leisure activity. This is about the uncontrolled and excessive draw to use shopping as a leisure activity, usually in an exclusive and overwhelming way. While activities such as window-shopping, visiting shops or spending time in commercial centres is a common and socially accepted desire activity, an addict is differentiated as one in whom this excessive attraction to purchase interferes with the normal development of life and damages their relationships with others, becoming an obsessive and uncontrolled activity.

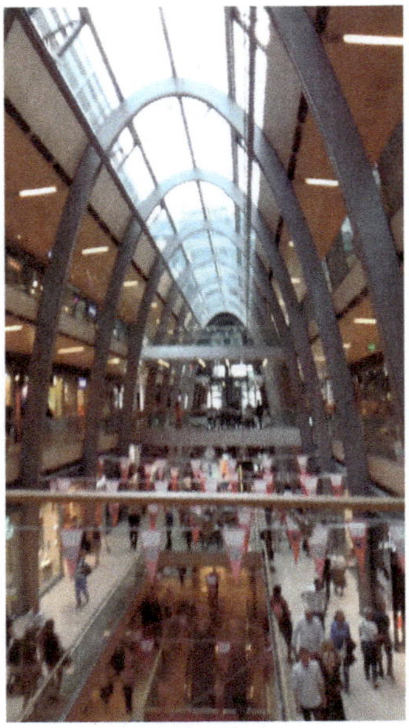

Huge malls become places to stay and ramble, show the use of shopping as a leisure activity.

Although shopping addiction and compulsive purchase are conceptually different, they are interrelated and both are manifestations of the same problem: the lack of self-control when buying and to restrain impulses. Shopping addiction is understood as the eagerness for constantly making new purchases of unnecessary or superfluous things. The concept of compulsive purchase is related to the psychological process which causes many people not to be able to control their impulses and wishes of buying, and subjects them to reflexion and evaluation before purchasing. A basic behavioural characteristic of people who have serious problems of consumer addiction is that their purchases are unnecessary and unsatisfactory. Addicts may feel pleasure or relief when they give in to the shopping wish, but regret it afterwards. In cases of people with severe problems of shopping addiction, this remorse can lead to very deep feelings of blame and discomfort.

Lack of economic self-control: this is the serious and permanent inability to adjust the habits of spending to the economic means of the individual. This is not about one's ordinary or unexpected spending making life difficult, but is an absolute inability to control the personal or family income in a rational way, and to discipline their buying, no matter how superfluous it is. A manifestation of this lack of control is usually the excessive use of indebtedness. The final result is the active or "guilty" over-indebtedness; this is which is derived from the improper behaviour of the consumer.

Impact on the General Population

The rate of people who have problems of shopping addiction is a very controversial matter, because the dividing line between pathological behaviours and those behaviours which, even if excessive, are socially accepted, is very difficult to determine. However, shopping addiction and other manifestations of the lack of self-control on spending are widespread problems which are constantly expanding. Studies using samples of the general population show that between 8% and 16% of the people have problems with excessive or uncontrolled purchases. Clinical studies give much lower figures, however, between 2% and 5%. According to the European Report on the programme for the prevention and treatment of personal problems related to consumer addiction, personal purchasing habits and over-indebtedness, 3% of European adults and 8% of European young people have a level of shopping addiction which could be considered as pathologic, that is, which seriously affects the life of the people who suffer from this. Other estimates for the prevalence of compulsive buying range from a low of 2 percent to 12 percent or more (in the U.S. population.). Most of people who have these problems neither receive nor ask for treatment. Those that ask for help only do it after years of suffering, when the addiction has caused very serious economic repercussion and has harmed the relationship with their family and social environment. For this reason and due to the lack of social consciousness about this problem, the unrecorded figure of people who suffer from these problems is very high. In addition to the severe cases of shopping addiction, an important part of consumers (between 30% and 50% of the population) have deficiencies with spending self-control or excessive purchases. According to the European Report, 33% of European adults and 46% of the European young people have minor or moderate problems with shopping addiction or lack of economic self-control.

Relationships with Other Disorders

The relationship of shopping addiction with other psychological disorders – especially with those regarding depression or anxiety - has been studied. This addiction has also been related with low self-esteem and with personality features such as impulsivity, materialism and hedonism.

Depression problems are the most frequent consequence in the most serious cases of shopping addiction. This is due to the fact that many consumers use shopping as a means to compensate or to face depressive states. Edwards (1992) in a research to study the influence of some personal variables in two groups, one of shopping addicts and another of non-addict consumers, came to the conclusion that depression is a trigger for shopping addiction problems. In agreement with this data, other researchers have pointed out the high incidence rate of depressive disorders among shopping addicts: Mc.Elloy (1994) placed at 25% the rate of addicts with depressive problems, Lejoyeux (1998) at 61%, and Black, Montaban and Gabel (1997) at 60%. More recent research shows that shopping addicts usually have feelings of leading an unsatisfactory and listless life, without any hope or excitement. In these cases, by means of purchase, the addicts seek for a way of escape, a satisfaction, even if momentary to compensate and to bear the depressive feelings.

Cole (1995) carried out research with a sample of 420 people and come to the conclusion that anxiety has an essential role in shopping addiction, as an antecedent or a triggering factor. In another study, Valence (1988) revealed that as the level of anxiety rises, the possibility of developing shopping addiction grows. Clinical research on the rate incidence of anxiety disorders in shopping addition also shows this relationship, although the percentage changes a lot: Shlosser (1994) 42%; McElroy (1994) 80%, and Christenson (1994) 50%. Research carried out by Garcés and Salcedo in 2005, based on a sample of 253 young people, concluded that the anxiety trait has a significant influence on shopping addiction but, by itself, is not determinant.

Population Differences

Gender

A higher rate of incidence of shopping addiction in women was pointed out in the first research works on the subject, so much so that it was considered a "women problem". Some researchers thought that this was a specifically female manifestation of problems of depression or obsessive-compulsive disorders. Others, from a psychoanalyst point of view, thought that it was a problem very similar to kleptomania and they related it to sexual repression to explain the high rate of incidence in women. Research carried out in the last century confirmed this difference although disagreeing on the scope. Other hypotheses have been stated to explain these differences. For example, people more easily develop addictions to behaviours they normally undertake and most home purchasing is still done by women. Since shopping is for many women one of their most usual activities, as obligation or as entertainment, it easily becomes an important mechanism of escape, facing other problems and ending up being an addiction. Another possible cause is that the most striking cases of shopping excesses are usually related to clothes, shoes, cosmetics and accessories, products which relate to physical appearance and are more frequently bought by women. The excessive purchase of other products such as electronic, computer or D.I.Y ones, accessories of cars, etc., that are frequently done by men usually goes unnoticed. This appraisal has been confirmed by research on different products bought by addicted women and men. Several studies (Flaber, O´Guin and Krych in1987, Scherhorn 1990, and McElroy in 1994),agree that women spend more on clothes, footwear, perfumes and, in general terms, men tend to spend more on sports equipment, car accessories and electronic products. The 1999 European Report established that women are drawn by activities like going shopping or window shopping, spending time in malls, escorting other people shopping. Moreover, they more frequently use shopping as a means of facing states of sadness, depression or downheartedness. However, the Report does not indicate significant differences between men and women related to economic self-control or impulsive purchase.

Age

Research carried out on people undergoing treatment, as well as on the general population has revealed a negative correlation between age and addiction. As the age of people increases there is a lower number of shopping addicts. This data was confirmed by the

1999 European Report. It must be noted that the age of diagnosis is much later than the age when the problems of addiction begin. Most addicts have the first symptoms of addiction in their twenties, but do not ask for help nor accept treatment until more than ten years afterwards. To explain the higher incidence of shopping addiction in young people, it has been shown that younger people have been born, and have grown up, in an increasingly consumerist society and they have endured the impact of publicity and marketing from birth. On the contrary, it is very unusual to find shopping addiction problems in people older than 65 years.

Different Theorical Approaches

Clinical approach: since ancient times, cases of people who bought in an uncontrolled way have been described, but the first relevant references to shopping addiction appear in the beginning of the twentieth century with Kraepelin and Bleuler. They analysed cases of people, usually women, who were not able to control their excess of purchasing and they considered this behaviour to be a symptom of other psychological diseases: depression, obsessive compulsive disorder, problems with control of impulses, etc. The clinical approach is also followed by the psychoanalytic theories that interpreted this behaviour as close to kleptomania and these would be manifestations of internal conflicts. Until the 1980s, this clinical approach was the predominant one in psychology and psychiatry. Shopping addiction was considered an individual disorder of impulse control or obsessive compulsive disorder, and its higher incidence rate in women and its relations with depression problems were emphasised.

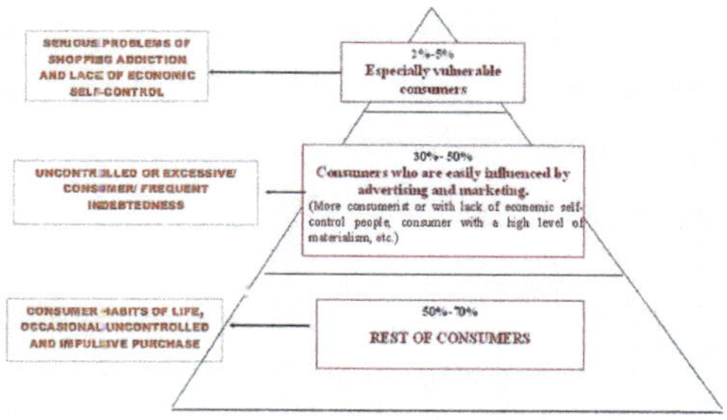

Psychosocial explanatory model of shopping addiction

Incidence rate of shopping addiction and other consumer problems of uncontrolled expending and indebtedness

(Garcés Prieto y Salcedo Aznal from EU statistics)

Psychosocial approach : Since the 1980s a significant increase in the number of people with important problems of lack of control in shopping and spending has been established. Given the fact that this increase was parallel with the spreading of the values and behaviour of the consumer society, these disorders started to be considered as an individual manifestation of a general social problem. A model taking this approach was one by Javier Garcés and Alejandro Saucedo, who regard shopping addiction as "the tip of the iceberg" that is, the most intense manifestation of a general problem which affects, to a greater or lesser extent, a great deal of the population. The behaviour differences between the average consumer and the shopping addict are more quantitative than qualitative. Advertising and commercial influences, which cause in some people serious problems of shopping addiction or excessive indebtedness, also contribute to excessive consumer behaviour in many others. This model is graphically described by the "consumerist pyramid". Another model is the one defended by Helga Ditmar, which could be classified as a mixed model, since she considers that shopping addiction problems are caused by the conjunction of two factors: a high level of materialism and a high discrepancy between the real self-concept (how the person sees themselves) and the ideal self-concept (how the person wishes to see themselves).

Shopping addiction as a drug-free addiction or as a social addiction: In this theoretical perspective, not incompatible with the previous approaches, shopping addiction is usually included among the so-called "drug-free addictions", such as addiction to gambling and, specifically, within a number of addictions grouped together as social addictions such as the addiction to Internet, video-games or mobile-phones.

Diagnosis

Since people buying more than they need is usual and accepted, even the most excessive behaviour takes a long time before being considered pathological. Shopping addiction generally manifests between 20–30 years old, but is not usually detected until several years after, when the addiction has led the person to ruin and bankrupt.

There are usually two stages in coping with the problem. First, people around the addict or the health or social services detect the problem and try to treat it. When, because of the seriousness of the case, it is not possible to solve it in this way, specialised professionals, such as psychologist or psychiatrics, take part. The diagnosis and evaluation of shopping addiction is based on the analysis of confirmed behaviours and their consequences. Specific tests or questionnaires, as the FACC-II (Questionnaire on the psychological aspects of consumer addiction, debt and personal spending habits) are also used. These specific questionnaires or tests are useful in the diagnosis and evaluation of shopping addiction problems, and to drive the therapies in a proper way. FACC-II is one of the most specific and widest. The Edwards Scale is another approach which measures the tendency to compulsively buy. All these resources, as well as personal interviews of the addict and people who surround them, reports and other documents, enable knowledge of when people buy, what they buy and the methods of payment used.

Treatment

Pharmacological Treatment

The inclusion of this problem in the obsessive-compulsive disorders and its relation with depression has led to some use of antidepressants as a treatment. Within antidepressant drugs, special attention has been paid to those related to serotonin, a brain neurotransmitter. This substance is supposed to be related to deficiencies in stimulus control, so that medicines like fluoxetine and fluvoxamine, which raise the level of serotonin in the brain, would be a pharmacological alternative to treat shopping addiction. Even though results are not conclusive, in the nineties some research was carried out which supported the effectiveness of tese treatments, at least in certain cases.

Behaviour Therapy

The treatment of shopping addiction – in contrast to other addictions as the gambling, alcohol or smoking - cannot seek to permanently remove the addicts from the behaviour. After therapy, they must be able to face consumer stimuli which surround them and maintain self-control. Because of this, the most usual therapies are behavioural ones., especially stimuli control and exposure and response prevention.

Guardianship

In the treatment of shopping addiction it is often very useful for other people – usually friends, relatives or educators -to help addicts control their expenses and impulsive purchases. In these cases, addicts have to accept that all their money, credit cards, bank accounts, etc, will be controlled by the guardian. This person becomes their "voluntary guardian". It is possible that the addict has also to accept not to go alone to stores and other limitations, even legal.

Self-registration Techniques

Self-registration techniques involve addicts noting down their activities to be able to remember and analyse them. This can range from a simple personal accountability of income and expenses, in the cases of minor economic lack of control, to a detailed diary of purchase, events and feelings, in the more serious cases of shopping addiction. Self-registration is useful to get clues about the behaviour, which could otherwise go unnoticed to the addicts themselves. Moreover, it is, in itself, a therapeutic means that helps addicts understand and reflect on their behaviour. These techniques are effective in improving economic self-control and avoiding impulsive purchase and are generally included, one way or another, in all programmes of treatment.

Self-help Groups and Group Therapy

Some experiences of self-help groups and group therapy have been carried out in a very similar way to those used in other addictions. Preliminary evidence suggests that group for compulsive shoppers colud be effective.

References

- Hofmann FG (1983). A Handbook on Drug and Alcohol Abuse: The Biomedical Aspects (2nd ed.). New York, USA: Oxford University Press. p. 329. ISBN 9780195030570

- Margolin, Arthur; et al. (2 January 2002). "Acupuncture for the treatment of cocaine addiction: A randomized controlled trial". The Journal of the American Medical Association. 287 (1)
- Mannfred A. Hollinger (19 October 2007). Introduction to Pharmacology, Third Edition. Abingdon: CRC Press. pp. 222–223. ISBN 978-1-4200-4742-4
- De Andrade, Marisa; Hastings, Gerald. "Tobacco Harm Reduction and Nicotine Containing Products" (PDF). Cancer Research UK. Cancer Research UK. p. 8. Retrieved 10 March 2016
- Levine, M. P.; Troiden, R. R. (1988). "The myth of sexual compulsivity". Journal of Sex Research. 25 (3): 347–363. doi:10.1080/00224498809551467
- Potter, Greg (2004). "Intensive therapy: Utilizing hypnosis in the treatment of substance abuse disorders". American Journal of Clinical Hypnosis. 47 (1): 21–28. PMID 15376606. doi:10.1080/00029157.2004.10401472
- D. B. Kandel (Ed.): Stages and Pathways of Drug Involvement: Examining the Gateway Hypothesis, Cambridge University Press, 2002, ISBN 978-0-521-78969-1, pp. 3-10
- USEPA (29 October 2008). "Nicotine; Notice of Receipt of Request to Voluntarily Cancel a Pesticide Registration". Federal Register: 64320–64322. Retrieved 8 April 2012
- Wadgave, U; Nagesh, L (2016). "Nicotine Replacement Therapy: An Overview.". International Journal of Health Sciences. 10 (3): 425–435. PMC 5003586. PMID 27610066
- Baselt, Randall Clint (2014). Disposition of Toxic Drugs and Chemicals in Man (10th ed.). Biomedical Publications. pp. 1452–6. ISBN 978-0-9626523-9-4
- Georgy Bakalkin (8 July 2008). "Alcoholism-associated molecular adaptations in brain neurocognitive circuits". Eurekalert.org. Retrieved 11 January 2012
- Giles, J. (2006). "No such thing as excessive levels of sexual behavior". Archives of Sexual Behavior. 35 (6): 641–642. PMID 17109229. doi:10.1007/s10508-006-9098-3
- Benowtz, N. L.; Herrera, B; Jacob p, 3rd (2004). "Mentholated Cigarette Smoking Inhibits Nicotine Metabolism". Journal of Pharmacology and Experimental Therapeutics. 310 (3): 1208–15. PMID 15084646
- Association, American Psychiatric (2013). Diagnostic and statistical manual of mental disorders : DSM-5. (5 ed.). Washington, D.C.: American Psychiatric Association. pp. 490–497. ISBN 9780890425541
- "Diagnostic Criteria for Alcohol Abuse and Dependence – Alcohol Alert No. 30-1995". Archived from the original on 27 March 2010. Retrieved 17 April 2010
- Li H Z, Rosenblood L (1994). "Exploring factors influencing alcohol consumption patterns among Chinese and Caucasians". Journal of Studies on Alcohol. 55 (4): 427. doi:10.15288/jsa.1994.55.427
- Diagnostic and statistical manual of mental disorders: DSM-IV. Washington, DC: American Psychiatric Association. 31 July 1994. ISBN 978-0-89042-025-6
- O'Connor PG (February 2012). "Amphetamines". Merck Manual for Health Care Professionals. Merck. Retrieved 8 May 2012
- Patrick TM, McBee ET, Hass HB (June 1946). "Synthesis of arylpropylamines; from allyl chloride". J. Am. Chem. Soc. 68: 1009–1011. PMID 20985610. doi:10.1021/ja01210a032

3

Substance Abuse and Disorders

Dependency on drugs that alter perception and consciousness of users is substance abuse. Mood changes, problems at work or school, change in behavior or changing in eating habits are some symptoms of substance abuse. Substance use disorder, opioid use disorder and amphetamine dependence are some topics explained in the following chapter.

Substance Abuse

Substance abuse, also known as drug abuse, is a patterned use of a drug in which the user consumes the substance in amounts or with methods which are harmful to themselves or others, and is a form of substance-related disorder. Widely differing definitions of drug abuse are used in public health, medical and criminal justice contexts. In some cases criminal or anti-social behavior occurs when the person is under the influence of a drug, and long term personality changes in individuals may occur as well. In addition to possible physical, social, and psychological harm, use of some drugs may also lead to criminal penalties, although these vary widely depending on the local jurisdiction.

Drugs most often associated with this term include: alcohol, cannabis, barbiturates, benzodiazepines, cocaine, methaqualone, opioids and some substituted amphetamines. The exact cause of substance abuse is not clear, with theories including one of two: either a genetic disposition which is learned from others, or a habit which if addiction develops, it manifests itself as a chronic debilitating disease.

In 2010 about 5% of people (230 million) used an illicit substance. Of these 27 million have high-risk drug use otherwise known as recurrent drug use causing harm to their health, psychological problems, or social problems or puts them at risk of those dangers. In 2015 substance use disorders resulted in 307,400 deaths, up from 165,000 deaths in 1990. Of these, the highest numbers are from alcohol use disorders at 137,500, opioid use disorders at 122,100 deaths, amphetamine use disorders at 12,200 deaths, and cocaine use disorders at 11,100.

Classification

Public Health Definitions

Public health practitioners have attempted to look at substance use from a broader perspective than the individual, emphasizing the role of society, culture, and availability.

Some health professionals choose to avoid the terms alcohol or drug "abuse" in favor of language they consider more objective, such as "substance and alcohol type problems" or "harmful/problematic use" of drugs. The Health Officers Council of British Columbia – in their 2005 policy discussion paper, *A Public Health Approach to Drug Control in Canada]* – has adopted a public health model of psychoactive substance use that challenges the simplistic black-and-white construction of the binary (or complementary) antonyms "use" vs. "abuse". This model explicitly recognizes a spectrum of use, ranging from beneficial use to chronic dependence.

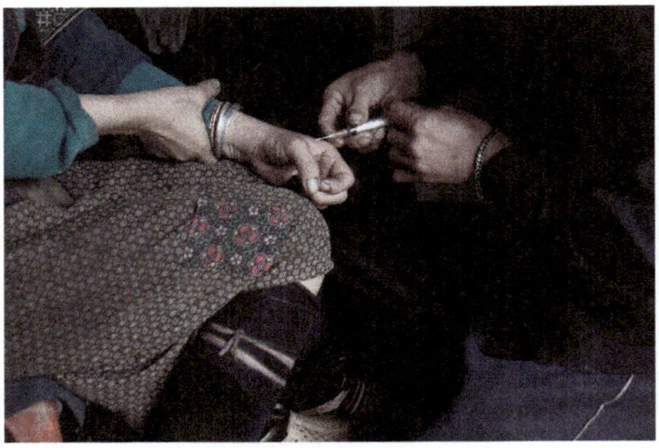

Drug users injecting heroin, an opiate

Medical Definitions

'Drug abuse' is no longer a current medical diagnosis in either of the most used diagnostic tools in the world, the American Psychiatric Association's Diagnostic and Statistical Manual of Mental Disorders (DSM), and the World Health Organization's International Statistical Classification of Diseases and ICRIS Medical organization Related Health Problems (ICD).

Substance abuse has been adopted by the DSM as a blanket term to include 10 separate classes of drugs, including alcohol; caffeine; cannabis; hallucinogens; inhalants; opioids; sedatives, hypnotics, and anxiolytics; stimulants; tobacco; and other substances. The ICD uses the term *Harmful use* to cover physical or psychological harm to the user from use.

Physical dependence, abuse of, and withdrawal from drugs and other miscellaneous substances is outlined in the DSM.

When an individual persists in use of alcohol or other drugs despite problems related to use of the substance, substance dependence may be diagnosed. Compulsive and repetitive use may result in tolerance to the effect of the drug and withdrawal symptoms when use is reduced or stopped.

However, other definitions differ; they may entail psychological or physical *dependence*, and may focus on treatment and prevention in terms of the social consequences of substance uses.

Drug Misuse

Drug misuse is a term used commonly when prescription medication with sedative, anxiolytic, analgesic, or stimulant properties are used for mood alteration or intoxication ignoring the fact that overdose of such medicines can sometimes have serious adverse effects. It sometimes involves drug diversion from the individual for whom it was prescribed.

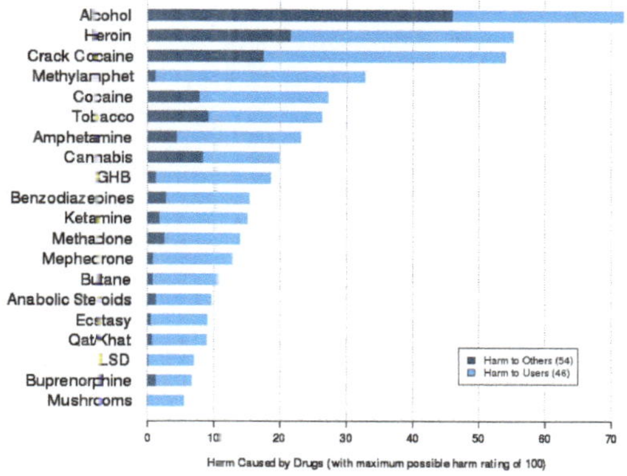

Legal drugs are not necessarily safer. A 2010 study asked drug-harm experts to rank various illegal and legal drugs. Alcohol was found to be the overall most dangerous drug.

Prescription misuse has been defined differently and rather inconsistently based on status of drug prescription, the uses without a prescription, intentional use to achieve intoxicating effects, route of administration, co-ingestion with alcohol, and the presence or absence of dependence symptoms. Chronic use of certain substances leads to a change in the central nervous system known as a 'tolerance' to the medicine such that more of the substance is needed in order to produce desired effects. With some substances, stopping or reducing use can cause withdrawal symptoms to occur, but this is highly dependent on the specific substance in question.

The rate of prescription drug use is fast overtaking illegal drug use in the United States. According to the National Institute of Drug Abuse, 7 million people were taking prescription drugs for nonmedical use in 2010. Among 12th graders, nonmedical prescription drug use is now second only to cannabis. "Nearly 1 in 12 high school seniors reported nonmedical use of Vicodin; 1 in 20 reported such use of OxyContin." Both of these drugs contain opioids.

Avenues of obtaining prescription drugs for misuse are varied: sharing between family and friends, illegally buying medications at school or work, and often "doctor shopping" to find multiple physicians to prescribe the same medication, without knowledge of other prescribers.

Increasingly, law enforcement is holding physicians responsible for prescribing controlled substances without fully establishing patient controls, such as a patient "drug contract." Concerned physicians are educating themselves on how to identify medication-seeking behavior in their patients, and are becoming familiar with "red flags" that would alert them to potential prescription drug abuse.

As a Value Judgment

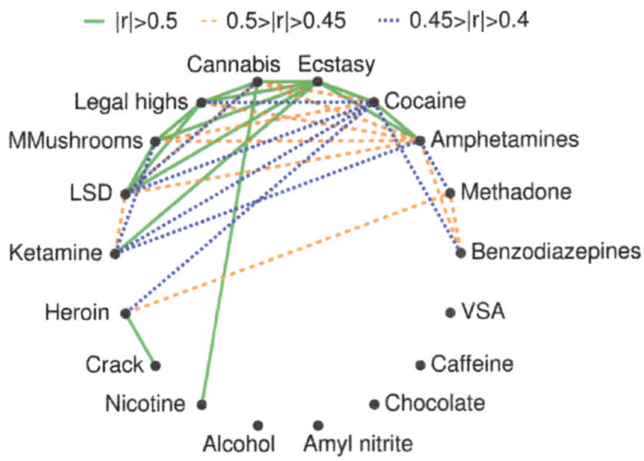

Correlations between usage of different drugs. Correlations between usage, within the previous decade, of 18 legal and illegal drugs: alcohol, amphetamines, amyl nitrite, benzodiazepine, cannabis, chocolate, cocaine, caffeine, crack, ecstasy, heroin, ketamine, legal highs, LSD, methadone, magic mushrooms (MMushrooms), nicotine and volatile substance abuse (VSA). Usage is defined as having used the drug at least once in the previous 10 years. Links indicate correlations with absolute values of Pearson correlation coefficient r above 0.4. Medium, strong, and very strong correlations are indicated by the colour of link.

Philip Jenkins suggests that there are two issues with the term "drug abuse". First, what constitutes a "drug" is debatable. For instance, GHB, a naturally occurring substance in the central nervous system is considered a drug, and is illegal in many countries, while nicotine is not officially considered a drug in most countries.

Second, the word "abuse" implies a recognized standard of use for any substance. Drinking an occasional glass of wine is considered acceptable in most Western countries, while drinking several bottles is seen as an abuse. Strict temperance advocates, who may or may not be religiously motivated, would see drinking even one glass as an abuse. Some groups even condemn caffeine use in any quantity. Similarly, adopting the view that any (recreational) use of cannabis or substituted amphetamines constitutes drug abuse implies a decision made that the substance is harmful, even in minute quantities. In the U.S., drugs have been legally classified into five categories, schedule I, II, III, IV, or V in the Controlled Substances Act. The drugs are classified on their deemed potential for abuse. Usage of some drugs is strongly correlated. For example, the consumption of seven illicit drugs (amphetamines, cannabis, cocaine, ecstasy, legal highs, LSD, and magic mushrooms) is correlated and the Pearson correlation coefficient $r>0.4$ in every pair of them; consumption of cannabis is strongly correlated ($r>0.5$) with usage of nicotine (tobacco), heroin is correlated with cocaine ($r>0.4$), methadone ($r>0.45$), and strongly correlated with crack ($r>0.5$).

Signs and Symptoms

Depending on the actual compound, drug abuse including alcohol may lead to health problems, social problems, morbidity, injuries, unprotected sex, violence, deaths, motor vehicle accidents, homicides, suicides, physical dependence or psychological addiction.

There is a high rate of suicide in alcoholics and other drug abusers. The reasons believed to cause the increased risk of suicide include the long-term abuse of alcohol and other drugs causing physiological distortion of brain chemistry as well as the social isolation. Another factor is the acute intoxicating effects of the drugs may make suicide more likely to occur. Suicide is also very common in adolescent alcohol abusers, with 1 in 4 suicides in adolescents being related to alcohol abuse. In the USA approximately 30% of suicides are related to alcohol abuse. Alcohol abuse is also associated with increased risks of committing criminal offences including child abuse, domestic violence, rapes, burglaries and assaults.

Drug abuse, including alcohol and prescription drugs, can induce symptomatology which resembles mental illness. This can occur both in the intoxicated state and also during the withdrawal state. In some cases these substance induced psychiatric disorders can persist long after detoxification, such as prolonged psychosis or depression after amphetamine or cocaine abuse. A protracted withdrawal syndrome can also occur with symptoms persisting for months after cessation of use. Benzodiazepines are the most notable drug for inducing prolonged withdrawal effects with symptoms sometimes persisting for years after cessation of use. Abuse of hallucinogens can trigger delusional and other psychotic phenomena long after cessation of use.

Cannabis may trigger panic attacks during intoxication and with continued use, it may cause a state similar to dysthymia. Researchers have found that daily cannabis use and the use of high-potency cannabis are independently associated with a higher chance of developing schizophrenia and other psychotic disorders.

Severe anxiety and depression are commonly induced by sustained alcohol abuse, which in most cases abates with prolonged abstinence. Even sustained moderate alcohol use may increase anxiety and depression levels in some individuals. In most cases these drug induced psychiatric disorders fade away with prolonged abstinence.

Impulsivity

Impulsivity is characterized by actions based on sudden desires, whims, or inclinations rather than careful thought. Individuals with substance abuse have higher levels of impulsivity, and individuals who use multiple drugs tend to be more impulsive. A number of studies using the Iowa gambling task as a measure for impulsive behavior found that drug using populations made more risky choices compared to healthy controls. There is a hypothesis that the loss of impulse control may be due to impaired inhibitory control resulting from drug induced changes that take place in the frontal cortex. The neurodevelopmental and hormonal changes that happen during adolescence may modulate impulse control that could possibly lead to the experimentation with drugs and may lead to the road of addiction. Impulsivity is thought to be a facet trait in the neuroticism personality domain (overindulgence/negative urgency) which is prospectively associated with the development of substance abuse.

Screening and Assessment

There are several different screening tools that have been validated for use with adolescents such as the CRAFFT Screening Test and in adults the CAGE questionnaire.

Treatment

Psychological

From the applied behavior analysis literature, behavioral psychology, and from randomized clinical trials, several evidenced based interventions have emerged: behavioral marital therapy, motivational Interviewing, community reinforcement approach, exposure therapy, contingency management They help suppress cravings and mental anxiety, improve focus on treatment and new learning behavioral skills, ease withdrawal symptoms and reduce the chances of relapse.

In children and adolescents, cognitive behavioral therapy (CBT) and family therapy currently has the most research evidence for the treatment of substance abuse problems. Well-established studies also include ecological family-based treatment and group CBT. These treatments can be administered in a variety of different formats, each of which has varying levels of research support Research has shown that what makes group CBT most effective is that it promotes the development of social skills, developmentally appropriate emotional regulatory skills and other interpersonal skills. A few integrated treatment models, which combines parts from various types of treatment, have also been seen as both well-established or probably effective. A study on maternal alcohol and drug use has shown that integrated treatment programs have produced significant results, resulting in higher negative results on toxicology screens. Additionally, brief school-based interventions have been found to be effective in reducing adolescent alcohol and cannabis use and abuse. Motivational interviewing can also be effective in treating substance use disorder in adolescents.

Alcoholics Anonymous and Narcotics Anonymous are one of the most widely known self-help organizations in which members support each other not to use alcohol. Social skills are significantly impaired in people suffering from alcoholism due to the neurotoxic effects of alcohol on the brain, especially the prefrontal cortex area of the brain. It has been suggested that social skills training adjunctive to inpatient treatment of alcohol dependence is probably efficacious, including managing the social environment.

Medication

A number of medications have been approved for the treatment of substance abuse. These include replacement therapies such as buprenorphine and methadone as well as antagonist medications like disulfiram and naltrexone in either short acting, or the newer long acting form. Several other medications, often ones originally used in other contexts, have also been shown to be effective including bupropion and modafinil. Methadone and buprenorphine are sometimes used to treat opiate addiction. These drugs are used as substitutes for other opioids and still cause withdrawal symptoms.

Antipsychotic medications have not been found to be useful. Acamprostate is a glutamatergic NMDA antagonist, which helps with alcohol withdrawal symptoms because alcohol withdrawal is associated with a hyperglutamatergic system.

Psychedelics, such as LSD and psilocin, may have anti-addictive properties.

Dual Diagnosis

It is common for individuals with drugs use disorder to have other psychological problems. The terms "dual diagnosis" or "co-occurring disorders," refer to having a mental health and substance use disorder at the same time. According to the British Association for Psychopharmacology (BAP), "symptoms of psychiatric disorders such as depression, anxiety and psychosis are the rule rather than the exception in patients misusing drugs and/or alcohol."

Individuals who have a comorbid psychological disorder often have a poor prognosis if either disorder is untreated. Historically most individuals with dual diagnosis either received treatment only for one of their disorders or they didn't receive any treatment all. However, since the 1980s, there has been a push towards integrating mental health and addiction treatment. In this method, neither condition is considered primary and both are treated simultaneously by the same provider.

Epidemiology

The initiation of drug and alcohol use is most likely to occur during adolescence, and some experimentation with substances by older adolescents is common. For example, results from 2010 Monitoring the Future survey, a nationwide study on rates of substance use in the United States, show that 48.2% of 12th graders report having used an illicit drug at some point in their lives. In the 30 days prior to the survey, 41.2% of 12th graders had consumed alcohol and 19.2% of 12th graders had smoked tobacco cigarettes. In 2009 in the United States about 21% of high school students have taken prescription drugs without a prescription. And earlier in 2002, the World Health Organization estimated that around 140 million people were alcohol dependent and another 400 million with alcohol-related problems.

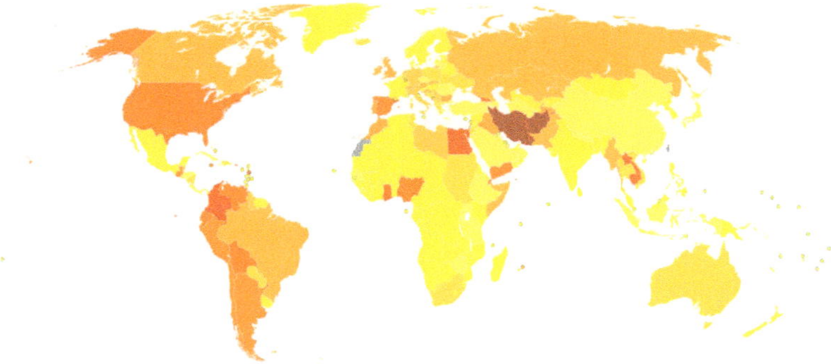

Disability-adjusted life year for drug use disorders per 100,000 inhabitants in 2004

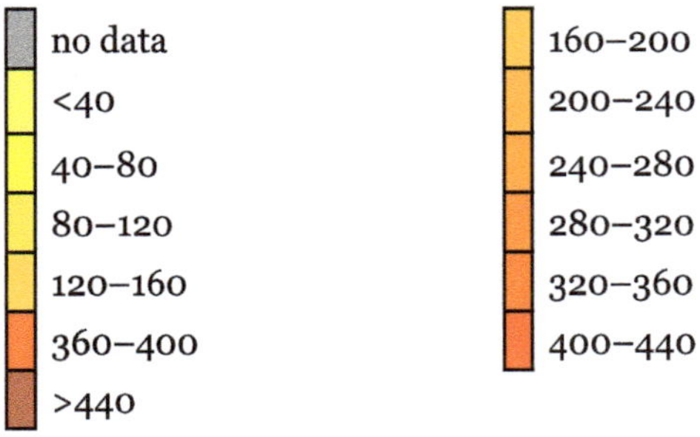

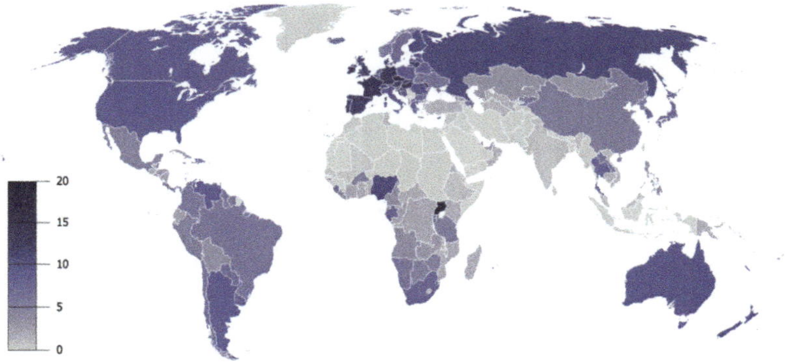

Total recorded alcohol per capita consumption (15+), in litres of pure alcohol

Studies have shown that the large majority of adolescents will phase out of drug use before it becomes problematic. Thus, although rates of overall use are high, the percentage of adolescents who meet criteria for substance abuse is significantly lower (close to 5%). According to BBC, "Worldwide, the UN estimates there are more than 50 million regular users of morphine diacetate (heroin), cocaine and synthetic drugs."

History

APA, AMA, and NCDA

In 1932, the American Psychiatric Association created a definition that used legality, social acceptability, and cultural familiarity as qualifying factors.

> as a general rule, we reserve the term drug abuse to apply to the illegal, non-medical use of a limited number of substances, most of them drugs, which have properties of altering the mental state in ways that are considered by social norms and defined by statute to be inappropriate, undesirable, harmful, threatening, or, at minimum, culture-alien."

In 1966, the American Medical Association's Committee on Alcoholism and Addiction defined abuse of stimulants (amphetamines, primarily) in terms of 'medical supervision':

> 'use' refers to the proper place of stimulants in medical practice; 'misuse' applies to the physician's role in initiating a potentially dangerous course of therapy; and 'abuse' refers to self-administration of these drugs without medical supervision and particularly in large doses that may lead to psychological dependency, tolerance and abnormal behavior.

In 1973, the National Commission on Marijuana and Drug Abuse stated:

> Drug abuse may refer to any type of drug or chemical without regard to its pharmacologic actions. It is an eclectic concept having only one uniform connotation: societal disapproval. The Commission believes that the term drug abuse must be deleted from official pronouncements and public policy dialogue. The term has no functional utility and has become no more than an arbitrary codeword for that drug use which is presently considered wrong.

DSM

The first edition of the American Psychiatric Association's Diagnostic and Statistical Manual of Mental Disorders (published in 1952) grouped alcohol and drug abuse under Sociopathic Personality Disturbances, which were thought to be symptoms of deeper psychological disorders or moral weakness. The third edition, published in 1980, was the first to recognize substance abuse (including drug abuse) and substance dependence as conditions separate from substance abuse alone, bringing in social and cultural factors. The definition of dependence emphasised tolerance to drugs, and withdrawal from them as key components to diagnosis, whereas abuse was defined as "problematic use with social or occupational impairment" but without withdrawal or tolerance.

In 1987, the DSM-IIIR category "psychoactive substance abuse," which includes former concepts of drug abuse is defined as "a maladaptive pattern of use indicated by continued use despite knowledge of having a persistent or recurrent social, occupational, psychological or physical problem that is caused or exacerbated by the use (or by) recurrent use in situations in which it is physically hazardous." It is a residual category, with dependence taking precedence when applicable. It was the first definition to give equal weight to behavioural and physiological factors in diagnosis. By 1988, the

DSM-IV defines substance dependence as "a syndrome involving compulsive use, with or without tolerance and withdrawal"; whereas substance abuse is "problematic use without compulsive use, significant tolerance, or withdrawal." Substance abuse can be harmful to your health and may even be deadly in certain scenarios. By 1994, The fourth edition of the Diagnostic and Statistical Manual of Mental Disorders (DSM) issued by the American Psychiatric Association, the DSM-IV-TR, defines substance dependence as "when an individual persists in use of alcohol or other drugs despite problems related to use of the substance, substance dependence may be diagnosed." followed by criteria for the diagnose

DSM-IV-TR defines substance abuse as:

- A. A maladaptive pattern of substance use leading to clinically significant impairment or distress, as manifested by one (or more) of the following, occurring within a 12-month period:
    1. Recurrent substance use resulting in a failure to fulfill major role obligations at work, school, or home (e.g., repeated absences or poor work performance related to substance use; substance-related absences, suspensions or expulsions from school; neglect of children or household)
    2. Recurrent substance use in situations in which it is physically hazardous (e.g., driving an automobile or operating a machine when impaired by substance use)
    3. Recurrent substance-related legal problems (e.g., arrests for substance-related disorderly conduct)
    4. Continued substance use despite having persistent or recurrent social or interpersonal problems caused or exacerbated by the effects of the substance (e.g., arguments with spouse about consequences of intoxication, physical fights)
- B. The symptoms have never met the criteria for Substance Dependence for this class of substance.

The fifth edition of the DSM (DSM-5), planned for release in 2013, is likely to have this terminology revisited yet again. Under consideration is a transition from the abuse/dependence terminology. At the moment, abuse is seen as an early form or less hazardous form of the disease characterized with the dependence criteria. However, the APA's 'dependence' term, as noted above, does not mean that physiologic dependence is present but rather means that a disease state is present, one that most would likely refer to as an addicted state. Many involved recognize that the terminology has often led to confusion, both within the medical community and with the general public. The American Psychiatric Association requests input as to how the terminology of this illness should be altered as it moves forward with DSM-5 discussion.

Society and Culture

Legal Approaches

Most governments have designed legislation to criminalize certain types of drug use. These drugs are often called "illegal drugs" but generally what is illegal is their unlicensed production, distribution, and possession. These drugs are also called "controlled substances". Even for simple possession, legal punishment can be quite severe (including the death penalty in some countries). Laws vary across countries, and even within them, and have fluctuated widely throughout history.

Attempts by government-sponsored drug control policy to interdict drug supply and eliminate drug abuse have been largely unsuccessful. In spite of the huge efforts by the U.S., drug supply and purity has reached an all-time high, with the vast majority of resources spent on interdiction and law enforcement instead of public health. In the United States, the number of nonviolent drug offenders in prison exceeds by 100,000 the total incarcerated population in the EU, despite the fact that the EU has 100 million more citizens.

Despite drug legislation (or perhaps because of it), large, organized criminal drug cartels operate worldwide. Advocates of decriminalization argue that drug prohibition makes drug dealing a lucrative business, leading to much of the associated criminal activity.

Cost

Policymakers try to understand the relative costs of drug-related interventions. An appropriate drug policy relies on the assessment of drug-related public expenditure based on a classification system where costs are properly identified.

Labelled drug-related expenditures are defined as the direct planned spending that reflects the voluntary engagement of the state in the field of illicit drugs. Direct public expenditures explicitly labeled as drug-related can be easily traced back by exhaustively reviewing official accountancy documents such as national budgets and year-end reports. Unlabelled expenditure refers to unplanned spending and is estimated through modeling techniques, based on a top-down budgetary procedure. Starting from overall aggregated expenditures, this procedure estimates the proportion causally attributable to substance abuse (Unlabelled Drug-related Expenditure = Overall Expenditure × Attributable Proportion). For example, to estimate the prison drug-related expenditures in a given country, two elements would be necessary: the overall prison expenditures in the country for a given period, and the attributable proportion of inmates due to drug-related issues. The product of the two will give a rough estimate that can be compared across different countries.

Europe

As part of the reporting exercise corresponding to 2005, the European Monitoring Centre for Drugs and Drug Addiction's network of national focal points set up in the 27 European Union (EU) Member States, Norway, and the candidates countries to the EU, were requested to identify labeled drug-related public expenditure, at the country level.

This was reported by 10 countries categorized according to the functions of government, amounting to a total of EUR 2.17 billion. Overall, the highest proportion of this total came within the government functions of Health (66%) (e.g. medical services), and Public Order and Safety (POS) (20%) (e.g. police services, law courts, prisons). By country, the average share of GDP was 0.023% for Health, and 0.013% for POS. However, these shares varied considerably across countries, ranging from 0.00033% in Slovakia, up to 0.053% of GDP in Ireland in the case of Health, and from 0.003% in Portugal, to 0.02% in the UK, in the case of POS; almost a 161-fold difference between the highest and the lowest countries for Health, and a 6-fold difference for POS. Why do Ireland and the UK spend so much in Health and POS, or Slovakia and Portugal so little, in GDP terms?

To respond to this question and to make a comprehensive assessment of drug-related public expenditure across countries, this study compared Health and POS spending and GDP in the 10 reporting countries. Results found suggest GDP to be a major determinant of the Health and POS drug-related public expenditures of a country. Labelled drug-related public expenditure showed a positive association with the GDP across the countries considered: $r = 0.81$ in the case of Health, and $r = 0.91$ for POS. The percentage change in Health and POS expenditures due to a one percent increase in GDP (the income elasticity of demand) was estimated to be 1.78% and 1.23% respectively.

Being highly income elastic, Health and POS expenditures can be considered luxury goods; as a nation becomes wealthier it openly spends proportionately more on drug-related health and public order and safety interventions.

UK

The UK Home Office estimated that the social and economic cost of drug abuse to the UK economy in terms of crime, absenteeism and sickness is in excess of £20 billion a year. However, the UK Home Office does not estimate what portion of those crimes are unintended consequences of drug prohibition (crimes to sustain expensive drug consumption, risky production and dangerous distribution), nor what is the cost of enforcement. Those aspects are necessary for a full analysis of the economics of prohibition.

United States

Year	Cost (billions of dollars)
1992	107
1993	111
1994	117
1995	125
1996	130
1997	134
1998	140
1999	151
2000	161
2001	170
2002	181

These figures represent overall economic costs, which can be divided in three major components: health costs, productivity losses and non-health direct expenditures.

- Health-related costs were projected to total $16 billion in 2002.
- Productivity losses were estimated at $128.6 billion. In contrast to the other costs of drug abuse (which involve direct expenditures for goods and services), this value reflects a loss of potential resources: work in the labor market and in household production that was never performed, but could reasonably be expected to have been performed absent the impact of drug abuse.

  Included are estimated productivity losses due to premature death ($24.6 billion), drug abuse-related illness ($33.4 billion), incarceration ($39.0 billion), crime careers ($27.6 billion) and productivity losses of victims of crime ($1.8 billion).
- The non-health direct expenditures primarily concern costs associated with the criminal justice system and crime victim costs, but also include a modest level of expenses for administration of the social welfare system. The total for 2002 was estimated at $36.4 billion. The largest detailed component of these costs is for state and federal corrections at $14.2 billion, which is primarily for the operation of prisons. Another $9.8 billion was spent on state and local police protection, followed by $6.2 billion for federal supply reduction initiatives.

According to a report from the Agency for Healthcare Research and Quality (AHRQ), Medicaid was billed for a significantly higher number of hospitals stays for Opioid drug overuse than Medicare or private insurance in 1993. By 2012, the differences were diminished. Over the same time, Medicare had the most rapid growth in number of hospital stays.

Special Populations

Immigrants and Refugees

Immigrant and refugees have often been under great stress, physical trauma and depression and anxiety due to separation from loved ones often characterize the pre-migration and transit phases, followed by "cultural dissonance," language barriers, racism, discrimination, economic adversity, overcrowding, social isolation, and loss of status and difficulty obtaining work and fears of deportation are common. Refugees frequently experience concerns about the health and safety of loved ones left behind and uncertainty regarding the possibility of returning to their country of origin. For some, substance abuse functions as a coping mechanism to attempt to deal with these stressors.

Immigrants and refugees may bring the substance use and abuse patterns and behaviors of their country of origin, or adopt the attitudes, behaviors, and norms regarding substance use and abuse that exist within the dominant culture into which they are entering.

Street Children

Street children in many developing countries are a high risk group for substance misuse, in particular solvent abuse. Drawing on research in Kenya, Cottrell-Boyce argues that "drug use amongst street children is primarily functional – dulling the senses against the hardships of life on the street – but can also provide a link to the support structure of the 'street family' peer group as a potent symbol of shared experience."

Musicians

In order to maintain high-quality performance, some musicians take chemical substances. Some musicians take drugs or alcohol to deal with the stress of performing. As a group they have a higher rate of substance abuse. The most common chemical substance which is abused by pop musicians is cocaine, because of its neurological effects. Stimulants like cocaine increase alertness and cause feelings of euphoria, and can therefore make the performer feel as though they in some ways 'own the stage'. One way in which substance abuse is harmful for a performer (musicians especially) is if the substance being abused is aspirated. The lungs are an important organ used by singers, and addiction to cigarettes may seriously harm the quality of their performance. Smoking causes harm to alveoli, which are responsible for absorbing oxygen.

Veterans

Substance abuse can be another contributing factor that affects physical and mental health of veterans. Substance abuse may also damage personal relationships families and lead to financial difficulty. There is evidence to suggest that substance abuse disproportionately affects the homeless veteran population. A 2015 Florida study compared causes of homelessness between veterans and non veteran populations in a self reporting questionnaire. The results from the study found that 17.8% of the homeless veteran participants attributed their homelessness to alcohol and drug related problems compared to just 3.7% of the non-veteran homeless group.

A 2003 study found that homelessness was associated with access to support from family/friends and services. However, this relationship was not true when comparing homeless participants who had a current substance-use disorders. The U.S. Department of Veterans Affairs provide a summary of treatment options for veterans with substance use disorder. For treatments that do not involve medication, they offer a therapeutic options that focused on finding outside support groups and "looking at how substance use problems may relate to other problems such as PTSD and depression".

Substance-related Disorder

Substance abuse, also known as drug abuse, is a patterned use of a substance (drug) in which the user consumes the substance in amounts or with methods which are harmful to themselves or others. The drugs used are often associated with levels of intoxication that alter judgment, perception, attention and physical control, not related with medical or therapeutic effects. It is often thought that the main abused substances are illegal drugs and alcohol; however it is becoming more common that prescription drugs and tobacco are a prevalent problem.

Substance-related disorders, including both substance dependence and substance abuse, can lead to large societal problems. It is found to be greatest in individuals ages 18–25, with a higher likelihood occurring in men compared to women, and urban residents compared to rural residents. On average, general medical facilities hold 20% of patients with substance-related disorders, possibly leading to psychiatric disorders later on. Over 50% of individuals with substance-related disorders will often have a "dual diagnosis," where they are diagnosed with the substance abuse, as well as a psychiatric diagnosis, the most common being major depression, personality disorder, anxiety disorders, and dysthymia.

Signs and Symptoms

Common symptoms include:

- Sudden changes in behaviour – may engage in secretive or suspicious behaviour
- Mood changes – anger towards others, paranoia and little care shown about themselves or their future
- Problems with work or school – lack of attendance

- Changes in eating and sleeping habits
- Changes in friendship groups and poor family relationships
- A sudden unexplained change in financial needs – leading to borrowing/stealing money

There are many more symptoms such as physical and psychological changes, though this is often dependent on which drug is being abused. It is, however, common that abusers will experience unpleasant withdrawal symptoms if the drug is taken away from them.

It is also reported that others have strong cravings even after they have not used the drug for a long period of time. This is called being "clean". To determine how the brain triggers these cravings, multiple tests have been done on mice. It is also now thought that these cravings can be explained by substance-related disorders as a subcategory of personality disorders as classified by the DSM-5.

Classification and Terminology

Substance-related disorders were originally subcategorized into "substance use disorders" (SUD) and "substance-induced disorders" (SID). Though DSM-IV makes a firm distinction between the two, SIDs often occur in the context of SUDs.

Substance-induced Disorders

Substance-induced disorders include medical conditions that can be directly attributed to the use of a substance. These conditions include intoxication, withdrawal, substance-induced delirium, substance-induced psychosis, and substance-induced mood disorders.

Substance use Disorders

Substance use disorders include substance abuse and substance dependence. In DSM-IV, the conditions are formally diagnosed as one or the other, but it has been proposed that DSM-V combine the two into a single condition called "Substance-use disorder".

Changes in Classification

The more recently published DSM-5 combined substance abuse and substance dependence into a single continuum; this is simply known as substance use disorder and requires more presenting symptoms before a diagnosis is made. It also considers each different substance as its own separate disorder, based upon the same basic criteria. It also distinguishes the difference between dependence and addictions as two separate disorders, not to be confused.

Potential Complications

There are many potential complications that can arise due to substance abuse such as severe physiological damage, psychological changes and social changes that are often not desirable.

Physiological damage is often the most obvious, observed as an abnormal condition affecting the body of an organism. For instance, there are several known alcohol-induced diseases (e.g. alcoholic hepatitis, alcoholic liver disease, alcoholic cardiomyopathy.) Substance abuse is also often associated with premature ageing, fertility complications, brain damage and a higher risk of infectious diseases due to a weakened immune system.

Long term abuse has been linked to personality changes such as depression, paranoia, anxiety which can be related to psychological disorders. It is often reported that substance abuse coincides with personality disorders, such as borderline personality disorder. It has also now been linked to severe brain damage leading to an inability to control behaviours, which could explain why many people who abuse substances go on to develop addictions.

Substance abuse is often regarded as negative in society and therefore those who engage in such behaviours can often be subject to social discrimination. The use of many drugs can lead to criminal convictions, whether the drug itself is illegal or abusers use unlawful methods to fund their substances. It is also more likely that someone will partake in criminal or anti-social behaviour when they are under the influence of a drug.

Epigenetics of Cocaine Addiction

Cocaine addiction is the compulsive use of cocaine despite adverse consequences. It arises through epigenetic modification (e.g., through HDAC, sirtuin, and G9a) and transcriptional regulation (primarily through ΔFosB's AP-1 complex) of genes in the nucleus accumbens.

Transcriptional and Epigenetic Mechanisms

Role of HDAC Inhibitors in Cocaine Addiction

Histone deacetylase inhibitors (HDAC inhibitors) have been implicated as a potential treatment for cocaine addicts. HDACs are enzymes that can deacetylate the histones associated with genes. This can activate genes for transcription. Several experiments have shown that inhibiting HDACs involved in histone H3K9 deacetylation reduces drug seeking behavior.

It has been known that epigenetic regulations, such as the methylation of H3K9, have a key role in the mechanism of addiction. Recent studies have shown that administering HDAC inhibitors can help reduce the craving for cocaine in rats. Trichostatin A (TsA) is an HDAC inhibitor associated with reduced cocaine-seeking behaviors; it inhibits HDAC classes 1, 3, 4, 6, and 10. Since this HDAC inhibitor has such a significant effect on cocaine-seeking behaviors, scientists have speculated about their ability to reduce a cocaine addict's risk of relapse in the rat model system during rehab.

After several tests in which rats were exposed to cocaine followed by either an HDAC inhibitor or a placebo, it was found that HDAC inhibitors had a significant effect on lowering cocaine-seeking behavior. This also suggests an epigenetic mechanism involved in HDAC chromatin regulation. The data is crucial to proving the hypothesis that trichostatin A can remodel chromatin structure and prevent behavioral changes following cocaine exposure. Tests also revealed that HDAC inhibitor administration can not only prevent addiction, but also helps reduce the risk of a relapse in cocaine addicts in the rat model system.

Role of HDAC5

As the previous findings suggest, chronic cocaine use caused both alterations in the chromatin remodeling activity of HDACs and drug seeking behavior. Renthal et al. focused specifically on the class II histone deacetylase, HDAC5, since it was known to have activity-dependent regulation in neurons. In fact, they found that HDAC5 was a central regulator of the actions of chronic cocaine use and contributed to the behavioral adaptations with its deacetylase activity. Chronic cocaine injections increased HDAC5 phosphorylation at Ser259 in the nucleus accumbens (NAc) within 30 minutes. This provides docking sites for 14-3-3 proteins, which mediate the export of HDAC5 out of the nucleus. They also found that CaMKII was necessary for depolarization-induced HDAC5 phosphorylation in NAc tissue, highlighting its role as a kinase for HDAC5. Experiments with mutant proteins and HDAC inhibitors suggested that HDAC5's action is mediated through its catalytic histone deacetylase domain. Rapid phosphorylation and the export of HDAC5 from the nucleus following cocaine use most likely leads to increased "pulses" of acetylation, targeted gene activation, and behavioral adaptations to long-term cocaine exposure.

The second set of experiments that Renthal et al. performed showed that chronic cocaine use induced upregulation of the NK_1 receptor protein in HDAC5 knockout mice, which is associated with hyperacetylation of H3 at the NK1R gene promoter. The NK1R gene promoter has been associated with enhanced response to cocaine reward, meaning HDAC5 in normal genomes may decrease cocaine reward with chronic cocaine exposure. They also found key pathways that were implicated in neural plasticity and reward behavior, which included DA receptor signaling, ATF2/CREB signaling, NF-κB, NFAT, cytoskeletal remodeling proteins, and ion channels. Their data implicated chromatin remodeling as a mechanism that drives altered gene activation and behavioral responses to cocaine. Using this they were able to conclude that within normal (wild type) genomes, the response to chronic cocaine includes phosphorylation of HDAC5 and export of the deacetylase out of the nucleus to activate downstream target genes. Between exposure and 24 hours after, HDAC5 returns to the cell nucleus to limit expression of these cocaine regulated genes by histone deacetylation. Their experiments with HDAC5 knockout mice lent additional support for this hypothesis. Since HDAC5 isn't there to limit the gene's expression, it begins to accumulate with repeated cocaine exposure, with the end result being increased sensitivity to cocaine reward.

Changes in Critical H3K9me3 Modifications

Modifications to histones such as methylations and acetylations can change gene expression patterns by activating or deactivating a region of DNA for transcription. The H3K9 position has been shown by several studies to be altered by chronic cocaine use.

Addictive behavior observed from long-term cocaine users can be due to changes of the gene expression profiles in the brain's reward circuitry. Most research has been focused on the active regions of the reward-related genes, but Maze et al. focuses at what happens to the heterochromatic regions. Maze et al. showed that heterochromatic regions in the nucleus accumbens (NAc), a major reward circuit in the brain, are significantly altered in the H3K9me3 position. Acute cocaine exposure leads to a rapid increase in H3K9me3 within half an hour and decreases back to normal levels within 24 hours. Chronic cocaine exposure leads to a slower increase in H3K9me3 within an hour (although it reaches the same level as acute by this time) and a 50% decrease from normal baseline levels within 24 hours. This chronic exposure was proposed to decrease heterochromatization (destabilization) within this brain region in patients given repeated cocaine exposure, which implies that the long-term addictive behaviors are affected by this epigenetic mark. They used ChIP-seq to provide supporting evidence that the H3K9me3 modification is mainly localized to intergenic regions. In these areas of the genome, 17 regions of repeat elements (SINEs, LINEs, LTRs, etc.) had significant H3K9me3 state changes in chronic cocaine exposure mouse models. They used quantitative PCR to determine that of these significant elements, the LINE-1 region showed a significant increase in expression levels. LINE-1 is a retrotransposon, so expressing it inappropriately can activate the transposon to insert itself within important genes and destabilizing the DNA. They conclude their findings by suggesting that LINE-1 retrotransposon insertions cause inappropriate or disrupted expression of genes leading to the addictive behavior.

Role of G9a in Changes to H3K9me2 Modification

Like Maze et al., studies by Covington et al. focused on histone modification in the nucleus accumbens. They suggest that the H3K9me2 modification in this area of the brain plays a role in the stress and depression pathway. Their idea was that cocaine modifies this epigenetic mark and that ths increases an addict's vulnerability to stress and depression, which leads to the addictive effects of these reagents. A methyltransferase, G9a, was found to have reduced expression in the nucleus accumbens in cocaine addicts, therefore causing reduced H3K9me2 levels. The genes that are unsilenced via acetylation of the heterochromatin abnormally express the genes involved in BDNF-TrkB-CREB signaling pathway. This causes enhanced phosphorylation of CREB downstream in the pathway. CREB causes enhanced acetylation and dis-regulation of the stress and depression signaling pathways.

Cocaine induces epigenetic changes that lead to neuronal morphology and behavioral changes. Most changes have to do with the disruption of heterochromatin caused by reduced levels of methylation on histones, namely H3K9. This decrease is mediated by the repression of G9a, a histone-lysine N-methyltransferase which is regulated by ΔFosB. ΔFosB is a cocaine-induced transcription factor that accumulates in the nucleus accumbens (NAc) and acts to repress G9a. When ΔFosB is overexpressed, G9a levels are reduced, and H3K9 dimethylation levels are reduced in the NAc. Maze et al. was interested in determining how the reduced levels affects the behavior of cocaine users. Several studies were done in rats and it was concluded that G9a overexpression, and thus the presence of H3K9 dimethylation, caused a decreased preference for cocaine in rats. Researchers then looked at the nuclear volume of rats exposed to cocaine and found that down-regulation of G9a increased the amount of dendritic spines in the nucleus accumbens leading to increased cocaine-seeking behavior.

It should be noted that only in the nucleus accumbens do G9a levels matter for cocaine addiction. Studies have been done in which G9a levels and H3K9me2 levels were changed in other areas of the brain, but these other locations had no effect on the cocaine-seeking behavior of rats.

Gene Expression Studies in the Mesolimbic Pathway

The role of sirtuin deacetylases have also been shown to play a role in mediating cocaine addiction. To determine their role, the two transcription factors previously mentioned, ΔFosB and CREB, first had to be analyzed. It has been previously stated that ΔFosB increases the cocaine-seeking behavior of users. This is because ΔFosB has a uniquely stable structure that allows it to persist and accumulate in the body. Unlike ΔFosB, CREB is responsible for reducing sensitivity to cocaine which causes negative symptoms during the withdrawal period. Each of these transcription factors increases the cocaine-seeking behavior of addicts. Once this connection between transcription factors had been established, the researchers were curious if other genes caused addictive behaviors too and explored the ones that were significant markers for cocaine addiction, one of which, was the sirtuin gene family. Sirtuins are Class III NAD-dependent histone deacetylases. Not only do sirtuins deacetylate histones, but are also responsible for the deacetylation of tubulin, p53, and NFKB. Several studies have explored the role sirtuins played in cocaine-seeking behavior. In one set of experiments, it was found that a significant increase in ΔFosB in the nucleus accumbens led to ΔFosB binding to the SIRT2 promoter. This increased binding caused acetylation of H3 which is associated with increased Sir2 mRNA. It was also found that the H3 acetylation induced by cocaine increased Sirt1 in the nucleus accumbens. Thus, repeated cocaine use causes an increase in both Sirt1 and Sirt2. Scientists were then interested in determining how increased Sirt1 and Sirt2 affected nuclear volume because it has been previously shown that repeated cocaine use does so. Scientists studying Sirt1 and Sirt2 have also found that these transcription factors led to increased nuclear volume. Therefore, it has been concluded that ΔFosB, CREB, Sirt1 and Sirt2 all play an integral role in cocaine-seeking behaviors.

Kumar et al. focused on how acute and chronic cocaine exposure affected the striatum, which is another area of the brain involved in the reward and locomotor pathways. To study the molecular actions of cocaine in this region, researchers studied the histone modifications of three different promoters: *cFos*, *BDNF*, and *Cdk5*. They saw that *cFos*, which is normally expressed immediately after neurons fire action potentials, had high levels of H4 acetylation within 30 minutes of a cocaine injection – but no histone modifications were seen with chronic cocaine use. These results suggested that this promoter is activated by acute cocaine use and possibly means that the neurons it regulates fire rapidly during acute cocaine exposure, yet are not affected by long-term use. *BDNF* has been implicated as a critical regulator in drug dependency, and Cdk5 is implicated in the regulation of cell proliferation genes. Both of these promoters were induced by chronic cocaine use (H3 hyperacetylation). Altering the natural acetylation states of these promoters in acute and chronic cocaine users altered the locomotor and reward responses to cocaine. This suggests that the behavioral activity observed by cocaine users can be attributed, in part, to the histone modifications at these promoter sites.

McClung et al. discuss the gene expression profiles of previously mentioned CREB and ΔFosB as they are involved in cocaine use. These transcription factors have been shown to play a role in the short-term and long-term adaptive changes in the brain. CREB has been implicated in learning, memory, and depression and enriched in cocaine users within the nucleus accumbens. CREB seems to upregulate many genes in its pathway within the reward regions of the brain and seems to reduce the rewarding effects of cocaine and leads to depressive-like behaviors instead. The gene expression changes by CREB are induced by short-term cocaine treatment and eventually go back to normal. They also focused on ΔFosB, which is in the family of FosB proteins. While most of these proteins have been implicated in short-term abuse gene expression changes, McClung et al. demonstrated that ΔFosB gene expression changes in the NAc were induced by short-term and long-term cocaine exposure. Short-term cocaine exposure lead to the same expression profiles of upregulated genes as CREB did creating the reduced rewarding effects seen. However, long-term exposure lead to a different expression profile leading to increased rewarding effects. They suggested that ΔFosB acts as a repressor and somehow interacts with the CREB pathway and indirectly leads to the same short-term effects seen, but over time, acts to upregulate genes within its own pathway leading to the increased rewarding effects. It is unknown how these two pathways interact, but they have shown that there is some overlap.

Modifications to the Gene Expression of Dopamine Receptor Pathways

Also involved in the CREB-Fos protein pathways is the dopamine D1 receptor (DRD1), expressed in neurons in the nucleus accumbens and caudate putamen regions. Zhang et al. focused on this receptor, as it is known to mediate the effects of cocaine. When stimulated, it increases cAMP levels, in turn leading to CREB activation. They had observed previous cocaine injections led to a direct increase in D1 receptor sensitivity. Through lines of D1 receptor mutant mice it had also been implicated in mediating both the locomotor sensation and rewarding effects of cocaine. Acute cocaine injections induced c-fos and CREB expression via D1 receptors and repeat cocaine administration, which associated with long lasting AP-1 transcription complexes containing ΔFosB. Persistent ΔFosB expression in D1 receptors in nucleus accumbens led to a significant increase in the locomotor-stimulating and rewarding effects of cocaine. Conversely, an increase of CREB was shown to decrease the rewarding effects of cocaine. Zhang et al. also used microarrays to identify specific genes induced by chronic cocaine use, which depend on a functional D1 receptor 24 hours after cocaine withdrawal. There were 109 genes identified that were either up or down regulated by 1.2 fold or more in the caudate putamen D1 receptor mutant mice after repeat injections. The expression of these genes was totally normal in mice with functional D1 receptors, suggesting chronic cocaine use had a direct influence on mediating these genes through a functional DRD1 receptor They found genes belonging to a number of functional groups, and chose six candidate genes from three of these functional groups to verify their differential expression in the caudate putamen. For each gene, researchers verified dependency of their expression on the D1 receptor after cocaine treatment using Trichostatin A or other receptor antagonists. Specifically, they focused on the genes encoding extracellular factors, receptors, modulators, and intracellular signaling molecules. These can be regulated by chronic cocaine treatment via D1 receptors, and all of the genes contain AP-1 transcriptional complex binding sites in their promoter regions. For extracellular signaling molecules, they looked at expression of the genes IGFBP6 and SDF1. Both of these were induced in the caudate putamen in wild type mice, but attenuated in the D1 receptor mutants. This suggests that IGFBP6 and SDF1 can be induced by repeat cocaine administration, and also that this interaction is partially dependent on a functional D1 receptor.

Direct Changes to Functional Groups

Zhang et al. had previously seen that chronic cocaine administration leads to increased dendritic branching and spine density on medium spine neurons and prefrontal cortex pyramidal neurons, which may contribute to cocaine-induced neuroadaptations. When investigating the genes that were receptors and modulators, they found that expression of the sigma 1 receptor and *RGS4* was not upregulated after repeat cocaine administration in DA D1 receptor mutants, suggesting functional dopamine D1 receptor is necessary for their induction. This receptor had been seen to modulate the rewarding effects of cocaine, and receptor antagonists had blocked the acute locomotor stimulating effect and lowered behavioral sensitization. Changes in the sigma 1 receptor have been shown to modulate dopamine release, so shifts in its expression can change the behavioral responses to cocaine with pre and post synaptic influences. They knew that *RGS4* proteins can modulate G-protein-coupled receptor function, and since *RGS4* levels can increase or decrease in response to D1/D2 receptor stimulation it could be involved in alterations of the signal transduction pathway after D1 receptor activation from repeat cocaine stimulation.

For the genes that encoded intracellular signaling molecules, Zhang et al. focused on the *Wrch1* gene. After experimentation researchers found *Wrch1* was upregulated by repeat cocaine injections in the caudate putamen in D1 receptor mutants. There was no change in wild type mice, leading them to believe that *Wrch1* may inhibit cocaine-induced and D1 receptor mediated behavioral changes. A key member of the Wnt signaling pathway, β-catenin, was thought to be induced by chronic cocaine administration (which had been true in the nucleus accumbens) but acute cocaine reduced expression in the caudate putamen whereas chronic cocaine injections decreased expression even in the NAc in D1 receptor mutants. This pathway influences Wrch1, so it can also influence cocaine-induced neuroadaptations. Lastly, they found that CaMKII-α was not upregulated as expected, and CD2 was downregulated in D1 receptor mutants after chronic treatment. These results suggest gene expression changes are definitely induced by chronic cocaine exposure via the D1 receptor and most at AP-1 binding sites.

Alterations in the Mesocorticolimbic System

Contrary to most studies focusing on the nucleus accumbens, Febo et al. suggested that the reward brain circuitry is not the only system involved in addictive behaviors. Previous knowledge has suggested that stimulants induce changes in gene expression in the main parts of mesolimbic circuitry (including the ventral tegmental area, ventral striatum/nucleus accumbens, and prefrontal cortex) and play a big role in development and maintenance of addicted state and chromatin remodeling. They applied this knowledge to investigate whether these gene expression changes are involved in cocaine related behavioral and molecular adaptations. They found unexpected patterns of brain activation in awake rats that were exposed to sodium butyrate, an HDAC inhibitor (or HDACi). An acute dose resulted in widespread BOLD (blood-oxygen-level dependent) activation in the forebrain and midbrain, but cocaine-induced activation was significantly attenuated after repeat exposure. Sodium butyrate co-treatment with cocaine restored pronounced BOLD activation after successive cocaine treatments. These suggest that the brain's initial response to repeat cocaine exposure triggers a desensitization mechanism which can be overturned by pretreatment with sodium butyrate. The neural circuitry for the epigenetic modifications contributing to cocaine sensitivity was not the limited to the mesocorticolimbic dopamine system ("reward system") as they expected. Instead, they saw corticolimbic circuitry (implicated in emotion and memory) had a bigger role in HDACi related alterations of reward behaviors. Evidence that HDACi-mediated enhancement of a stimulant's sensitizing effects is context specific, and involves associative learning.

Treatment

As of May 2014, there is no effective approved pharmacotherapy for cocaine addiction. HDAC inhibitors have been implicated as a potential treatment for cocaine addiction.

Cognitive behavioral therapy is currently the most effective clinical treatment for psychostimulant addiction in general.

Drug Overdose

The term drug overdose (or simply overdose or OD) describes the ingestion or application of a drug or other substance in quantities greater than are recommended or generally practiced. An overdose may result in a toxic state or death.

Classification

The word "overdose" implies that there is a common safe dosage and usage for the drug; therefore, the term is commonly only applied to drugs, not poisons, though even poisons are harmless at a low enough dosage. Drug overdoses are sometimes caused intentionally to commit suicide, parasuicide or as self-harm, but many drug overdoses are accidental, the result of intentional or unintentional misuse of medication. Intentional misuse leading to overdose can include using prescribed or unprescribed drugs in excessive quantities in an attempt to produce euphoria.

Usage of illicit drugs of unexpected purity, in large quantities, or after a period of drug abstinence can also induce overdose. Cocaine users who inject intravenously can easily overdose accidentally, as the margin between a pleasurable drug sensation and an overdose is small. Unintentional misuse can include errors in dosage caused by failure to read or understand product labels. Accidental overdoses may also be the result of over-prescription, failure to recognize a drug's active ingredient, or unwitting ingestion by children. A common unintentional overdose in young children involves multi-vitamins containing iron. Iron is a component of the hemoglobin molecule in blood, used to transport oxygen to living cells. When taken in small amounts, iron allows the body to replenish hemoglobin, but in large amounts it causes severe pH imbalances in the body. If this overdose is not treated with chelation therapy, it can lead to death or permanent coma. The term 'overdose' is often misused as a descriptor for adverse drug reactions or negative drug interactions due to mixing multiple drugs simultaneously.

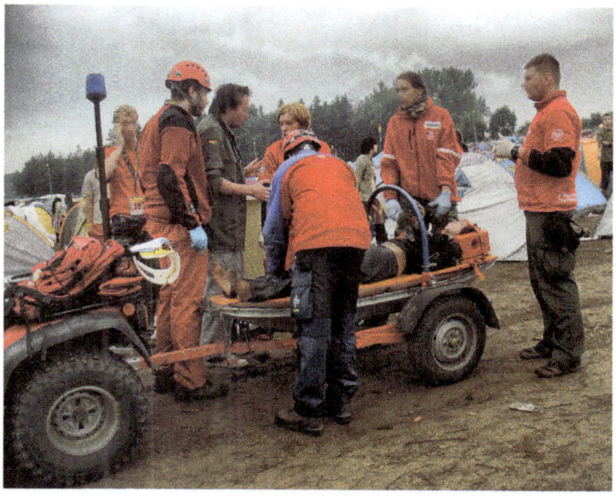

A music fan who has had a drug overdose at the Woodstock Music Festival is strapped into a wheeled cot by paramedics.

Signs and Symptoms

Toxidrome							
Symptoms	**BP**	**HR**	**RR**	**Temp**	**Pupils**	**bowel sounds**	**diaphoresis**
anticholinergic	~	up	~	up	dilated	down	down
cholinergic	~	~	unchanged	unchanged	constricted	up	up
opioid	down	down	down	down	constricted	down	down
sympathomimetic	up	up	up	up	dilated	up	up
sedative-hypnotic	down	down	down	down	~	down	down

Signs and symptoms of an overdose vary depending on the drug or toxin exposure. The symptoms can often be divided into differing toxidromes. This can help one determine what class of drug or toxin is causing the difficulties.

Symptoms of opioid overdoses include slow breathing, heart rate and pulse. Opioid overdoses can also cause pinpoint pupils, and blue lips and nails due to low levels of oxygen in the blood. A person experiencing an opioid overdose might also have muscle spasms, seizures and decreased consciousness. A person experiencing an opiate overdose usually will not wake up even if their name is called or if they are shaken vigorously.

Causes

The drugs or toxins that are most frequently involved in overdose and death (grouped by ICD-10):

- Acute alcohol intoxication (F10)
    - Ethyl alcohol
    - Methanol poisoning
    - Ethylene glycol poisoning
- Opioid overdose (F11)
- Among sedative-hypnotics (F13)
    - Barbiturate overdose (T42.3)
    - Benzodiazepine overdose (T42.4)
    - Uncategorized sedative-hypnotics (T42.6)
        - Ethchlorvynol (Placidyl)
        - GHB
        - Glutethimide (Doriden)
        - Methaqualone
        - Ketamine (T41.2)
- Among Stimulants (F14-F15)
    - Cocaine overdose (T40.5)
    - Amphetamine overdose (T43.6)
    - Methamphetamine (T43.6)
- Among Tobacco (F17)
    - Nicotine (T65.2)
- Among Poly drug use (F19)
    - Drug "cocktails" (Speedballs)
- Medications
    - Aspirin poisoning (T39.0)
    - Acetaminophen poisoning (Alone or mixed with Oxycodone)
    - Paracetamol toxicity (T39.1)

- Tricyclic antidepressant overdose (T43.0)
- Vitamin poisoning

- Pesticide poisoning (T60)
  - Organophosphate poisoning
  - DDT

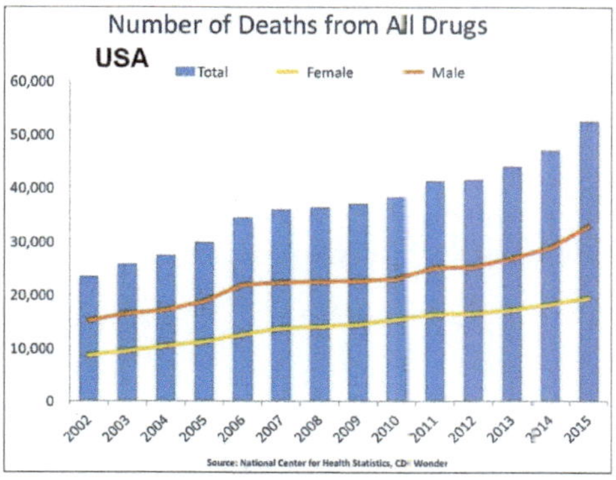

Timeline of number of yearly U.S. overdose deaths from all drugs.

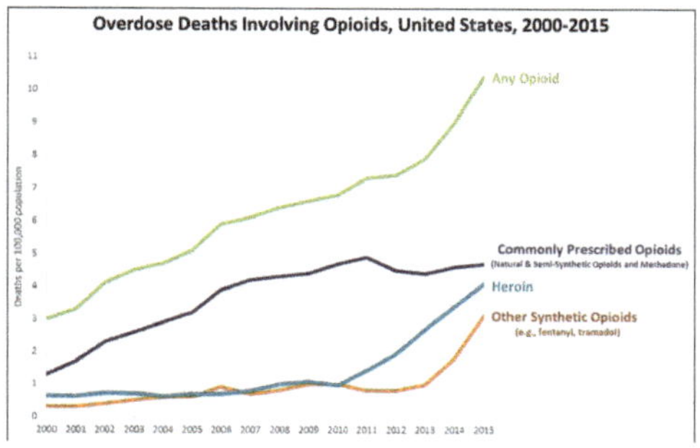

Overdose Deaths Involving Opioids, United States, 2000-2015. Deaths per 100,000 population.

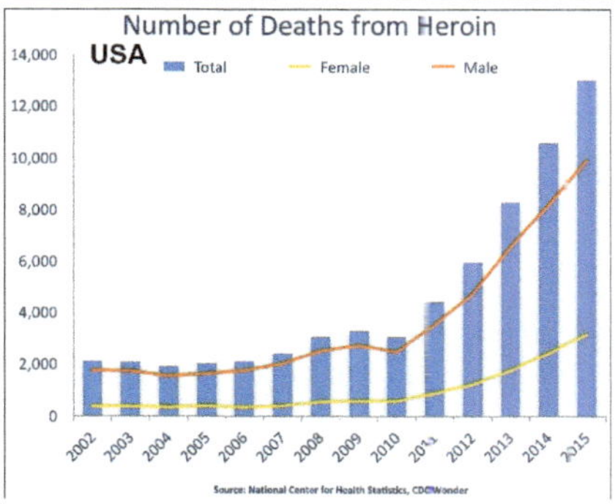

Timeline of number of yearly U.S. overdose deaths involving heroin.

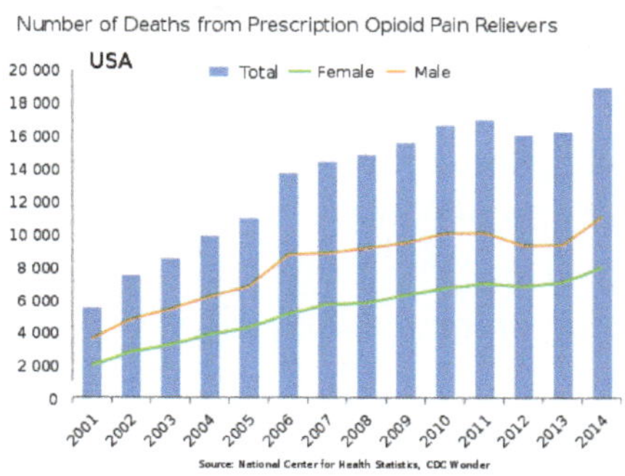

Timeline of number of yearly U.S. overdose deaths involving prescription opioid pain relievers.

Diagnosis

The substance that has been taken may often be determined by asking the person. However, if they will not, or cannot, due to an altered level of consciousness, provide this information, a search of the home or questioning of friends and family may be helpful.

Examination for toxidromes, drug testing, or laboratory test may be helpful. Other laboratory test such as glucose, urea and electrolytes, paracetamol levels and salicylate levels are typically done. Negative drug-drug interactions have sometimes been misdiagnosed as an acute drug overdose, occasionally leading to the assumption of suicide.

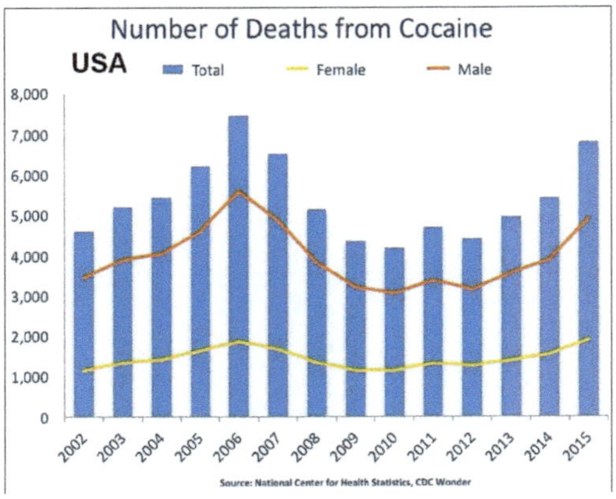

Timeline of number of yearly U.S. overdose deaths involving cocaine.

Prevention

The distribution of naloxone to injection drug users and other opioid drug users decreases the risk of death from overdose. The Centers for Disease Control and Prevention (CDC) estimates that U.S. programs for drug users and their caregivers prescribing take-home doses of naloxone and training on its utilization are estimated to have prevented 10,000 opioid overdose deaths. Healthcare institution-based naloxone prescription programs have also helped reduce rates of opioid overdose in the U.S. state of North Carolina, and have been replicated in the U.S. military. Nevertheless, scale-up of healthcare-based opioid overdose interventions is limited by providers' insufficient knowledge and negative attitudes towards prescribing take-home naloxone to prevent opioid overdose. Programs training police and fire personnel in opioid overdose response using naloxone have also shown promise in the US.

Management

Stabilization of the victim's airway, breathing, and circulation (ABCs) is the initial treatment of an overdose. Ventilation is considered when there is a low respiratory rate or when blood gases show the person to be hypoxic. Monitoring of the patient should continue before and throughout the treatment process, with particular attention to temperature, pulse, respiratory rate, blood pressure, urine output, electrocardiography (ECG) and O_2 saturation. Poison control centers and medical toxicologists are available in many areas to provide guidance in overdoses to both physicians and the general public.

Antidotes

Specific antidotes are available for certain overdoses. For example, Naloxone is the antidote for opiates such as heroin or morphine. Similarly, benzodiazepine overdoses may be effectively reversed with flumazenil. As a nonspecific antidote, activated charcoal is frequently recommended if available within one hour of the ingestion and the ingestion is significant. Gastric lavage, syrup of ipecac, and whole bowel irrigation are rarely used.

Epidemiology and Statistics

47,055 drug overdose deaths occurred in the United States in 2014. Since 2000, the drug overdose death rate has gone from 6.2 per 100,000 persons in 2000 to 14.7 per 100,000 in 2014.

The National Center for Health Statistics report that 19,250 people died of accidental poisoning in the U.S. in the year 2004 (8 deaths per 100,000 population).

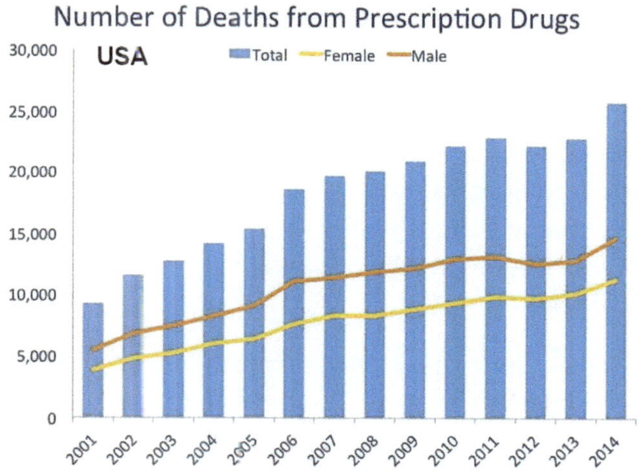

Timeline of number of yearly U.S. overdose deaths involving prescription drugs.

In 2008 testimony before a Senate subcommittee, Leonard J. Paulozzi, a medical epidemiologist at the Centers for Disease Control and Prevention stated that in 2005 more than 22,000 American lives were lost due to overdoses, and the number is growing rapidly. Paulozzi also testified that all available evidence suggests that unintentional overdose deaths are related to the increasing use of prescription drugs, especially opioid painkillers. However, the vast majority of overdoses are also attributable to alcohol. It is very rare for a victim of an overdose to have consumed just one drug. Most overdoses occur when drugs are ingested in combination with alcohol. According to the Centers for Disease Control and Prevention, every day in the U.S., 44 people die of drug overdoses.

Drug overdose was the leading cause of injury death in 2013. Among people 25 to 64 years old, drug overdose caused more deaths than motor vehicle traffic crashes. There were 43,982 drug overdose deaths in the United States in 2013. Of these, 22,767 (51.8%) were related to prescription drugs.

The 22,767 deaths relating to prescription drug overdose in 2013, 16,235 (71.3%) involved opioid painkillers, and 6,973 (30.6%) involved benzodiazepines. Drug misuse and abuse caused about 2.5 million emergency department (ED) visits in 2011. Of these, more than 1.4 million ED visits were related to prescription drugs. Among those ED visits, 501,207 visits were related to anti-anxiety and insomnia medications, and 420,040 visits were related to opioid analgesics.

Substance use Disorder

Substance use disorder (SUD), also known as drug use disorder, is a condition in which the use of one or more substances leads to a clinically significant impairment or distress. Although the term *substance* can refer to any physical matter, 'substance' in this context is limited to psychoactive drugs. Addiction and dependence are components of a substance use disorder and addiction represents the most severe form of the disorder.

SUD refers to the overuse of, or dependence on, a drug leading to effects that are detrimental to the individual's physical and mental health, or the welfare of others. SUD is characterized by a pattern of continued pathological use of a medication, non-medically indicated drug or toxin, which results in repeated adverse social consequences related to drug use, such as failure to meet work, family, or school obligations, interpersonal conflicts, or legal problems.

There are on-going debates as to the exact distinctions between substance abuse and substance dependence, but current practice standard distinguishes between the two by defining substance dependence in terms of physiological and behavioral symptoms of substance use, and substance abuse in terms of the social consequences of substance use. In the DSM-5 substance use disorder replaced substance abuse and substance dependence.

In 2010 about 5% of people (230 million) used an illicit substance. Of these 27 million have high-risk drug use otherwise known as recurrent drug use causing harm to their health, psychological problems, or social problems or puts them at risk of those dangers. In 2015 substance use disorders resulted in 307,400 deaths, up from 165,000 deaths in 1990. Of these, the highest numbers are from alcohol use disorders at 137,500, opioid use disorders at 122,100 deaths, amphetamine use disorders at 12,200 deaths, and cocaine use disorders at 11,100.

Definitions

Substance abuse may lead to addiction, substance dependence, or both. Medically, physiologic dependence requires the development of tolerance leading to withdrawal symptoms. Both abuse and dependence are distinct from addiction which involves a compulsion to continue using the substance despite the negative consequences, and may or may not involve chemical dependency. Dependence often implies abuse, but abuse frequently occurs without dependence, particularly when an individual first begins to abuse a substance. Dependence involves physiological processes while substance abuse reflects a complex interaction between the individual, the abused substance and society.

Substance abuse is sometimes used as a synonym for drug abuse, drug addiction, and chemical dependency, but actually refers to the use of substances in a manner outside sociocultural conventions. All use of controlled drugs and all use of other drugs in a manner not dictated by convention (e.g. according to physician's orders or societal norms) is abuse according to this definition; however there is no universally accepted definition of substance abuse.

The physical harm for twenty drugs was compared in an article in the Lancet. Physical harm was assigned a value from 0 to 3 for acute harm, chronic harm and intravenous harm. Shown is the mean physical harm. Not shown, but also evaluated, was the social harm.

Substance use may be better understood as occurring on a spectrum from beneficial to problematic use. This conceptualization moves away from the ill-defined binary antonyms of "use" vs. "abuse" towards a more nuanced, public health-based understanding of substance use.

The Diagnostic and Statistical Manual of Mental Disorders (DSM-IV TR) describes physical dependence, abuse of, and withdrawal from drugs and other substances. It does not use the word 'addiction' at all. It has instead a section about substance dependence:

"Substance dependence When an individual persists in use of alcohol or other drugs despite problems related to use of the substance, substance dependence may be diagnosed. Compulsive and repetitive use may result in tolerance to the effect of the drug and withdrawal symptoms when use is reduced or stopped. This, along with Substance Abuse are considered Substance Use Disorders"

Signs and Symptoms

The DSM definition of addiction can be boiled down to compulsive use of a substance (or engagement in an activity) despite ongoing negative consequences. The medical community makes a distinction between physical dependence (characterized by symptoms of physical withdrawal symptoms, like tremors and sweating) and psychological dependence (emotional-motivational withdrawal symptoms). Physical dependence is simply needing a substance to function. Humans are all physically dependent upon oxygen, food and water. A drug can cause physical dependence and not psychological dependence (for example, some blood pressure medications, which can produce fatal withdrawal symptoms if not tapered) and some can cause psychological dependence without physical dependence (the withdrawal symptoms associated with cocaine are all psychological, there is no associated vomiting or diarrhea as there is with opiate withdrawal).

There are several different screening tools that have been validated for use with adolescents such as the CRAFFT and adults such as the CAGE.

Addiction

Physical Dependency

Physical dependence on a substance is defined by the appearance of characteristic physical withdrawal symptoms when the substance is suddenly discontinued. Opiates, benzodiazepines, barbiturates, alcohol and nicotine induce physical dependence. On the other hand, some categories of substances share this property and are still not considered addictive: cortisone, beta blockers and most antidepressants are examples.

Some substances induce physical dependence or physiological tolerance - but not addiction — for example many laxatives, which are not psychoactive; nasal decongestants, which can cause rebound congestion if used for more than a few days in a row; and some antidepressants, most notably venlafaxine, paroxetine and sertraline, as they have quite short half-lives, so stopping them abruptly causes a more rapid change in the neurotransmitter balance in the brain than many other antidepressants. Many non-addictive prescription drugs should not be suddenly stopped, so a doctor should be consulted before abruptly discontinuing them.

The speed with which a given individual becomes addicted to various substances varies with the substance, the frequency of use, the means of ingestion, the intensity of pleasure or euphoria, and the individual's genetic and psychological susceptibility. Some people may exhibit alcoholic tendencies from the moment of first intoxication, while most people can drink socially without ever becoming addicted. Opioid dependent individuals have different responses to even low doses of opioids than the majority of people, although this may be due to a variety of other factors, as opioid use heavily stimulates pleasure-inducing neurotransmitters in the brain. Nonetheless, because of these variations, in addition to the adoption and twin studies that have been well replicated, much of the medical community is satisfied that addiction is in part genetically moderated. That is, one's genetic makeup may regulate how susceptible one is to a substance and how easily one may become attached to a pleasurable routine.

Eating disorders are complicated pathological mental illnesses and thus are not the same as addictions described. Eating disorders, which some argue are not addictions at all, are driven by a multitude of factors, most of which are highly different from the factors behind addictions described. It has been reported, however, that patients with eating disorders can successfully be treated with the same non-pharmacological protocols used in patients with chemical addiction disorders.

Gambling is another potentially addictive behavior with some biological overlap. Conversely gambling urges have emerged with the administration of Mirapex (pramipexole), a dopamine agonist.

The obsolete term physical addiction is deprecated, because of its connotations. In modern pain management with opioids physical dependence is nearly universal. High-quality, long-term studies are needed to better delineate the risks and benefits of chronic opiate use.

Psychological Dependency

Psychological dependency on a substance is defined by the appearance of emotional-motivational withdrawal symptoms (e.g., anxiety, irritability, anhedonia, depressed mood, restlessness, etc.) when the substance is suddenly discontinued. Psychological dependence is not unique to substances; for example, separation anxiety occurs in young children when they lack exposure to individuals to whom they're emotionally attached.

Causes

Risk Factors

As demonstrated by the chart below, numerous studies have examined factors which mediate substance abuse or dependence. In these examples, the predictor variables lead to the mediator which in turn leads to the outcome, which is always substance abuse or dependence. For example, research has found that being raised in a single-parent home can lead to increased exposure to stress and that increased exposure to stress, not being raised in a single-parent home, leads to substance abuse or dependence. The following are some, but by no means all, of the possible mediators of substance abuse.

Predictor Variables	Mediator Variables	Outcome Variable
Single-parent Home	Exposure to Stress, Association w/ Deviant Peers	Substance Abuse or Dependence
Child Abuse/Neglect	PTSD symptoms, Stressful Life Events, Criminal Behavior	Substance Abuse or Dependence
Parental Substance Abuse Witnessing Violence	Physical/Sexual Abuse Delinquency Status	Substance Abuse or Dependence

As demonstrated by the chart below, numerous studies have examined factors which moderate substance abuse or dependence. In these examples, the moderator variable impacts the level to which the strength of the relationship varies between a given predictor variable and the outcome of substance abuse or dependence. For example, there is a significant relationship between psychobehavioral risk factors, such as tolerance of deviance, rebelliousness, achievement, perceived drug risk, familism, family church attendance and other factors, and substance abuse and dependence. That relationship is moderated by familism which means that the strength of the relationship is increased or decreased based on the level of familism present in a given individual.

Predictor Variables	Moderator Variables	Outcome Variable
Psychobehavioral Risk	Familism Family Church Attendance	Substance Abuse or Dependence
Victimization Effects	Race/Ethnicity Physical/Sexual Abuse	Substance Abuse or Dependence
Family History of Alcoholism	Gender	Substance Abuse or Dependence

Examples of mediators and moderators can be found in several empirical studies. For example, Pilgrim et al.'s hypothesized mediation model posited that school success and time spent with friends mediated the relationship between parental involvement and risk-taking behavior with substance use (2006). More specifically, the relationship between parental involvement and risk-taking behavior is explained via the interaction with third variables, school success and time spent with friends. In this example, increased parental involvement led to increased school success and decreased time with friends, both of which were associated with decreased drug use. Another example of mediation involved risk-taking behaviors. As risk-taking behaviors increased, school success decreased and time with friends increased, both of which were associated with increased drug use. A second example of a mediating variable is depression. In a study by Lo and Cheng (2007), depression was found to mediate the relationship between childhood maltreatment and subsequent substance abuse in adulthood. In other words, childhood physical abuse is associated with increased depression, which in turn, in associated with increased drug and alcohol use in young adulthood. More specifically, depression helps to explain how childhood abuse is related to subsequent substance abuse in young adulthood.

A third example of a mediating variable is an increase of externalizing symptoms. King and Chassin (2008) conducted research examining the relationship between stressful life events and drug dependence in young adulthood. Their findings identified problematic externalizing behavior on subsequent substance dependency. In other words, stressful life events are associated with externalizing symptoms, such as aggression or hostility, which can lead to peer alienation or acceptance by socially deviant peers, which could lead to increased drug use. The relationship between stressful life events and subsequent drug dependence however exists via the presence of the mediation effects of externalizing behaviors.

An example of a moderating variable is level of cognitive distortion. An individual with high levels of cognitive distortion might react adversely to potentially innocuous events, and may have increased difficulty reacting to them in an adaptive manner (Shoal & Giancola, 2005). In their study, Shoal and Giancola investigated the moderating effects of cognitive distortion on adolescent substance use. Individuals with low levels of cognitive distortion may be more apt to choose more adaptive methods of coping with social problems, thereby potentially reducing the risk of drug use. Individuals with high levels of cognitive distortions, because of their increased misperceptions and misattributions, are at increased risk for social difficulties. Individuals may be more likely to react aggressively or inappropriately, potentially alienating themselves from their peers, thereby putting them at greater risk for delinquent behaviors, including substance use and abuse. In this study, social problems are a significant risk factor for drug use when moderated by high levels of cognitive distortions.

Mechanisms

Addiction

ΔFosB, a gene transcription factor, has been identified as playing a critical role in the development of an addiction. Overexpression of ΔFosB in the nucleus accumbens is necessary and sufficient for many of the neural adaptations seen in drug addiction; it has been implicated in addictions to alcohol, cannabinoids, cocaine, nicotine, phenylcyclidine, and substituted amphetamines as well as addictions to natural rewards such as sex, exercise, and food. Moreover, reward cross-sensitization between amphetamine and sexual activity, a property in which exposure to one increases in the desire for both, has been shown to occur preclinically and clinically as a dopamine dysregulation syndrome; ΔFosB expression is required for this cross-sensitization effect, which intensifies with the level of ΔFosB expression.

Dependence

Upregulation of the cyclic adenosine monophosphate (cAMP) signal transduction pathway by cAMP response element binding protein (CREB), a gene transcription factor, in the nucleus accumbens is a common mechanism of psychological dependence among several classes of drugs of abuse. Upregulation of the same pathway in the locus coeruleus is also a mechanism responsible for certain aspects of opioid-induced physical dependence.

Increased brain-derived neurotrophic factor (BDNF) signaling in the ventral tegmental area (VTA) has been shown to mediate opiate-induced withdrawal symptoms via downregulation of insulin receptor substrate 2 (IRS2), protein kinase B (AKT), and mechanistic target of rapamycin complex 2 (mTORC2). As a result of downregulated signaling through these proteins, opiates cause VTA neuronal hyperexcitability and shrinkage (specifically, the size of the neuronal soma is reduced). It has been shown that when an opiate-naive person begins using opiates in concentrations that induce euphoria, BDNF signaling increases in the VTA.

Management

Addiction Severity Index

Some medical systems, including those of at least 15 states of the United States, refer to an Addiction Severity Index to assess the severity of problems related to substance use. According to DARA Thailand, the index assesses potential problems in seven categories: medical, employment/support, alcohol, other drug use, legal, family/social, and psychiatric.

Detoxification

Early treatment of acute withdrawal often includes medical detoxification, which can include doses of anxiolytics or narcotics to reduce symptoms of withdrawal. An experimental drug, ibogaine, is also proposed to treat withdrawal and craving.

Neurofeedback therapy has shown statistically significant improvements in numerous researches conducted on alcoholic as well as mixed substance abuse population. In chronic opiate addiction, a surrogate drug such as methadone is sometimes offered as a form of opiate replacement therapy. But treatment approaches universal focus on the individual's ultimate choice to pursue an alternate course of action.

Tailoring Treatment

Therapists often classify patients with chemical dependencies as either interested or not interested in changing.

Treatments usually involve planning for specific ways to avoid the addictive stimulus, and therapeutic interventions intended to help a client learn healthier ways to find satisfaction. Clinical leaders in recent years have attempted to tailor intervention approaches to specific influences that affect addictive behavior, using therapeutic interviews in an effort to discover factors that led a person to embrace unhealthy, addictive sources of pleasure or relief from pain.

Treatments		
Behavioral pattern	***Intervention***	***Goals***
Low self-esteem, anxiety, verbal hostility	Relationship therapy, client centered approach	Increase self-esteem, reduce hostility and anxiety
Defective personal constructs, ignorance of interpersonal means	Cognitive restructuring including directive and group therapies	Insight
Focal anxiety such as fear of crowds	Desensitization	Change response to same cue
Undesirable behaviors, lacking appropriate behaviors	Aversive conditioning, operant conditioning, counter conditioning	Eliminate or replace behavior
Lack of information	Provide information	Have client act on information
Difficult social circumstances	Organizational intervention, environmental manipulation, family counseling	Remove cause of social difficulty
Poor social performance, rigid interpersonal behavior	Sensitivity training, communication training, group therapy	Increase interpersonal repertoire, desensitization to group functioning
Grossly bizarre behavior	Medical referral	Protect from society, prepare for further treatment
Adapted from: *Essentials of Clinical Dependency Counseling*, Aspen Publishers		

From the applied behavior analysis literature and the behavioral psychology literature, several evidenced-based intervention programs have emerged (1) behavioral marital therapy (2) community reinforcement approach (3) cue exposure therapy and (4) contingency management strategies. In addition, the same author suggests that social skills training adjunctive to inpatient treatment of alcohol dependence is probably efficacious.

Epidemiology

In 2013 drug use disorders resulted in 127,000 deaths up from 53,000 in 1990. The highest number of deaths are from opioid use disorders at 51,000. Alcohol use disorders resulted in an addition 139,000 deaths.

About 10.6% of Americans with substance use disorder seek treatment, and 40-60% of those people relapse within a year.

Legality

Most countries have legislation which brings various drugs and drug-like substances under the control of licensing systems. Typically this legislation covers any or all of the opiates, substituted amphetamines, cannabinoids, cocaine, barbiturates, hallucinogens (tryptamines, LSD, phencyclidine, and psilocybin) and a variety of more modern synthetic drugs, and unlicensed production, supply or possession may be a criminal offense.

Usually, however, drug classification under such legislation is not related simply to addictiveness. The substances covered often have very different addictive properties. Some are highly prone to cause physical dependency, whilst others rarely cause any form of compulsive need whatsoever.

Also, although the legislation may be justifiable on moral grounds to some, it can make addiction or dependency a much more serious issue for the individual. Reliable supplies of a drug become difficult to secure as illegally produced substances may have contaminants. Withdrawal from the substances or associated contaminants can cause additional health issues and the individual becomes vulnerable to both criminal abuse and legal punishment. Criminal elements that can be involved in the profitable trade of such substances can also cause physical harm to users.

Opposition to Common Views

Thomas Szasz denies that addiction is a psychiatric problem. In many of his works, he argues that addiction is a choice, and that a drug addict is one who simply prefers a socially taboo substance rather than, say, a low risk lifestyle. In *Our Right to Drugs*, Szasz cites the biography of Malcolm X to corroborate his economic views towards addiction: Malcolm claimed that quitting cigarettes was harder than shaking his heroin addiction. Szasz postulates that humans always have a choice, and it is foolish to call someone an "addict" just because they prefer a drug induced euphoria to a more popular and socially welcome lifestyle.

Professor John Booth Davies at the University of Strathclyde has argued in his book *The Myth of Addiction* that "people take drugs because they want to and because it makes sense for them to do so given the choices available" as opposed to the view that "they are compelled to by the pharmacology of the drugs they take." He uses an adaptation of attribution theory (what he calls the theory of functional attributions) to argue that the statement "I am addicted to drugs" is functional, rather than veridical. Stanton Peele has put forward similar views.

Opioid use Disorder

Opioid use disorder is a medical condition characterized by a problematic pattern of opioid use that causes clinically significant impairment or distress. It often includes a strong desire to use opioids, increased tolerance to opioids, and withdrawal syndrome when opioids are abruptly discontinued. Addiction and dependence are components of a substance use disorder and addiction represents the most severe form of the disorder. Opioid dependence can manifest as physical dependence, psychological dependence, or both.

Opioids include substances such as morphine, heroin, codeine and oxycodone. These can be bought illegally or prescribed. The diagnosis of opioid use disorder is often based on criteria by the American Psychiatric Association in the DSM-5. These include a preoccupation with a desire to obtain and take opioids, as well as using more than intended despite social and professional consequences due to these behaviors.

Opioid use disorder can be treated with opioid replacement therapy using methadone or buprenorphine. Being on such treatment reduces the risk of death. Additionally, individuals with opioid use disorder may benefit from twelve-step programs, other peer support, and support from mental health professionals such as individual or group therapy. Naloxone is useful for the treatment of opioid overdose.

In 2013 opioid use disorders affects about 0.4% of people. About 16 million people have been affected at one point in time. It resulted in 122,000 deaths worldwide in 2015, up from 18,000 deaths in 1990. In the United States in 2015 there were 33,000 deaths due to drug overdose involving opioids. Of those 33,000 deaths, about 15,000 were from prescribed opioids and 13,000 from heroin.

Signs and Symptoms

Signs and symptoms include:

- Drug seeking behavior
- Multiple prescriptions from different providers

- Increased use over time
- Opioid cravings
- Multiple medical complications from drug use (HIV/AIDS, hospitalizations, abscesses)
- Legal or social ramifications secondary to drug use
- Withdrawal symptoms
- Constipation

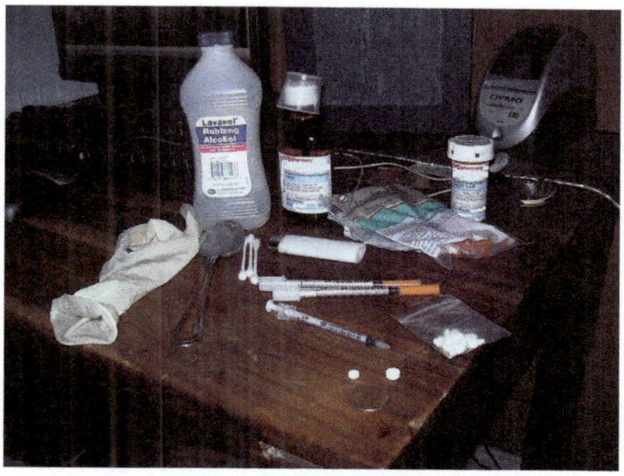

Material used for intravenous injection of opiates

Withdrawal

Symptoms of withdrawal from opiates include:

Early Symptoms

- Altered perception of temperature (hot/cold flashes)
- Agitation
- Anxiety
- Change in libido (abnormally high or low)
- Dehydration
- Fatigue
- Muscle aches
- Mental fog or confusion

- Lack of motivation
- Increased tearing
- Insomnia
- Restless legs
- Runny nose
- Sweating
- Yawning
- Skin-crawling

Late Symptoms

- Abdominal cramping
- Sneezing
- Diarrhea
- Dilated pupils
- Goose bumps
- Nausea
- Vomiting

Opioid Intoxication

Signs and symptoms of opioid intoxication include:

- Decreased perception of pain
- Euphoria
- Confusion
- Desire to sleep
- Nausea
- Constipation

Opioid Overdose

Signs and symptoms of opioid overdose include, but are not limited to:

- Pin-point pupils may occur. Patient presenting with dilated pupils may still be suffering an opioid overdose.
- Decreased heart rate
- Decreased body temperature
- Decreased breathing
- Altered level of consciousness. People may be unresponsive or unconscious.
- Pulmonary edema (fluid accumulation in the lungs)
- Shock
- Death

Cause

Most people who have an opioid use disorder have at least one other psychiatric co-morbidity. Opioid use disorder can develop as a result of self-medication, though this is controversial. Scoring systems have been derived to assess the likelihood of opiate addiction in chronic pain patients.

According to position papers on the treatment of opioid dependence published by the United Nations Office on Drugs and Crime and the World Health Organization, care providers should not treat opioid use disorder as the result of a weak character or will. Additionally, detoxification alone does not constitute adequate treatment.

Mechanism

Addiction

Addiction is a brain disorder characterized by compulsive drug use despite adverse consequences. Addiction is a component of a substance use disorder and represents the most severe form of the disorder.

Overexpression of the gene transcription factor "ΔFosB" in the nucleus accumbens plays a crucial role in the development of an addiction to opioids and other addictive drugs by sensitizing drug reward and amplifying compulsive drug-seeking behavior. Like other addictive drugs, overuse of opiates leads to increased ΔFosB expression in the nucleus accumbens. Opiates affect dopamine neurotransmission in the nucleus accumbens via the disinhibition of dopaminergic pathways as a result of inhibiting the GABA-based projections to the ventral tegmental area (VTA) from the rostromedial tegmental nucleus (RMTg), which negatively modulate dopamine neurotransmission. In other words, opiates inhibit the projections from the RMTg to the VTA, which in turn disinhibits the dopaminergic pathways that project from the VTA to the nucleus accumbens and elsewhere in the brain.

Neuroimaging has shown functional and structural alterations in the brain. A 2017 study showed that chronic intake of opiate, such as heroin, may cause long-term effect in the orbitofrontal area (OFC), which is essential for regulating reward-related behaviors, emotional responses, and anxiety. Moreover, neuroimaging and neuropsychological studies demonstrated dysregulation of circuits associated with emotion, stress and high impulsivity.

Dependence

Drug dependence is an adaptive state associated with a withdrawal syndrome upon cessation of repeated exposure to a stimulus (e.g., drug intake). Dependence is a component of a substance use disorder. Opioid dependence can manifest as physical dependence, psychological dependence, or both.

Increased brain-derived neurotrophic factor (BDNF) signaling in the ventral tegmental area (VTA) has been shown to mediate opiate-induced withdrawal symptoms via downregulation of insulin receptor substrate 2 (IRS2), protein kinase B (AKT), and mechanistic target of rapamycin complex 2 (mTORC2). As a result of downregulated signaling through these proteins, opiates cause VTA neuronal hyperexcitability and shrinkage (specifically, the size of the neuronal soma is reduced). It has been shown that when an opiate-naive person begins using opiates in concentrations that induce euphoria, BDNF signaling increases in the VTA.

Upregulation of the cyclic adenosine monophosphate (cAMP) signal transduction pathway by cAMP response element binding protein (CREB), a gene transcription factor, in the nucleus accumbens is a common mechanism of psychological dependence among several classes of drugs of abuse. Upregulation of the same pathway in the locus coeruleus is also a mechanism responsible for certain aspects of opioid-induced physical dependence.

Opioid Receptors

A genetic basis for the efficacy of opioids in the treatment of pain has been demonstrated for a number of specific variations; however, the evidence for clinical differences in opioid effects is ambiguous. The pharmacogenomics of the opioid receptors and their endogenous ligands have been the subject of intensive activity in association studies. These studies test broadly for a number of phenotypes, including opioid dependence, cocaine dependence, alcohol dependence, methamphetamine dependence/psychosis, response to naltrexone treatment, personality traits, and others. Major and minor variants have been reported for every receptor and ligand coding gene in both coding sequences, as well as regulatory regions. Newer approaches shift away from analysis of specific genes and regions, and are based on an unbiased screen of genes across the entire genome, which have no apparent relationship to the phenotype in question. These GWAS studies yield a number of implicated genes, although many of them code for seemingly unrelated proteins in processes such as cell adhesion, transcriptional regulation, cell structure determination, and RNA, DNA, and protein handling/modifying.

Currently, there are no specific pharmacogenomic dosing recommendations for opioids due to a lack of clear evidence connecting genotype to drug effect, toxicity, or likelihood of dependence.

118A>G variant

While over 100 variants have been identified for the opioid mu-receptor, the most studied mu-receptor variant is the non-synonymous 118A>G variant, which results in functional changes to the receptor, including lower binding site availability, reduced mRNA levels, altered signal transduction, and increased affinity for beta-endorphin. In theory, all of these functional changes would reduce the impact of exogenous opioids, requiring a higher dose to achieve the same therapeutic effect. This points to a potential for a greater addictive capacity in these individuals who require higher dosages to achieve pain control. However, evidence linking the 118A>G variant to opioid dependence is mixed, with associations shown in a number of study groups, but negative results in other groups. One explanation for the mixed results is the possibility of other variants which are in linkage disequilibrium with the 118A>G variant and thus contribute to different haplotype patterns that more specifically associate with opioid dependence.

Non-opioid Receptor Genes

The preproenkephalin gene, PENK, encodes for the endogenous opiates that modulate pain perception, and are implicated in reward and addiction. (CA) repeats in the 3' flanking sequence of the PENK gene was associated with greater likelihood of opiate dependence in repeated studies. Variability in the MCR2 gene, encoding melanocortin receptor type 2 has been associated with both protective effects and increased susceptibility to heroin addiction. The CYP2B6 gene of the cytochrome P450 family also mediates breakdown of opioids and thus may play a role in dependence and overdose.

Diagnosis

The DSM-5 guidelines for diagnosis of opioid use disorder require that the individual has significant impairment or distress related to opioid uses. In order to make the diagnosed two or more of eleven criteria must be present in a given year:

1. More opioids are taken than intended
2. The individual is unable to decrease the amount of opioids used
3. Large amounts of time are spent trying to obtain opioids, use opioids, or recover from taking them

4. The individual has cravings for opioids
5. Difficulty fulfilling professional duties at work or school
6. Continued use of opioids leading to social and interpersonal consequences
7. Decreased social or recreational activities
8. Using opioids despite it being physically dangerous settings
9. Continued use despite opioids worsening physical or psychological health (i.e. depression, constipation)
10. Tolerance
11. Withdrawal

Prevention

There are efforts to decrease the number of opioids prescribed in an effort to decrease opioid use disorder and deaths related to opioid use.

Opioid Related Deaths

The use of naloxone, an opioid receptor antagonist, can reduce the risk of death due to an opioid overdose. Naloxone kits are recommended for laypersons who may witness an opioid overdose, for individuals with large prescriptions for opioids, those in substance use treatment programs, or who have been recently released from incarceration.

Management

Opioid use disorders require long-term treatment and care with the goal of reducing health risks for the consumer, reducing criminal behaviour, and improving the long-term physical and psychological condition of the addicted person. Most strategies aim ultimately to reduce drug use and lead to abstinence.

No single treatment works for everyone, so several strategies have been developed including therapy and drugs.

Detox programs are rarely a good solution, and people often relapse after going through them, but it is an important first step.

As of 2013 in the US, there was a significant increase of prescription opioid abuse compared to illegal opiates like heroin. This development has also implications for the prevention, treatment and therapy of opioid dependence.

Medications

Opioid replacement therapy (ORT), also called opioid substitution therapy or opioid maintenance therapy, involves replacing an opioid, such as heroin, with a longer acting but less euphoric opioid. Commonly used drugs for ORT are methadone or buprenorphine which are taken under medical supervision.

The driving principle behind ORT is the program's capacity to facilitate a resumption of stability in the user's life, while the patient experiences reduced symptoms of drug withdrawal and less intense drug cravings; a strong euphoric effect is not experienced as a result of the treatment drug. In some countries (not the US, or Australia), regulations enforce a limited time period for people on ORT programs that conclude when a stable economic and psychosocial situation is achieved. (Patients suffering from HIV/AIDS or Hepatitis C are usually excluded from this requirement.) In practice, 40-65% of patients maintain complete abstinence from opioids while receiving opioid replacement therapy and 70-95% are able to reduce their use significantly. Along with this is a concurrent elimination or reduction in medical (improper diluents, non-sterile injecting equipment), psychosocial (mental health, relationships), and legal (arrest and imprisonment) issues that can arise from the use of illegal opioids. Clonidine or lofexidine can help treat the symptoms of withdrawal.

ORT has proven to be the most effective treatment for improving the health and living condition of people experiencing problematic illegal opiate use or dependence, including mortality reduction and overall societal costs, such as the economic loss from drug-related crime and healthcare expenditure. Opioid Replacement Therapy is endorsed by the World Health Organization, United Nations Office on Drugs and Crime and UNAIDS as being effective at reducing injection, lowering risk for HIV/AIDS, and promoting adherence to antiretroviral therapy. Currently, 55 countries worldwide use methadone replacement therapy, while some countries such as Russia do not offer it.

Methadone

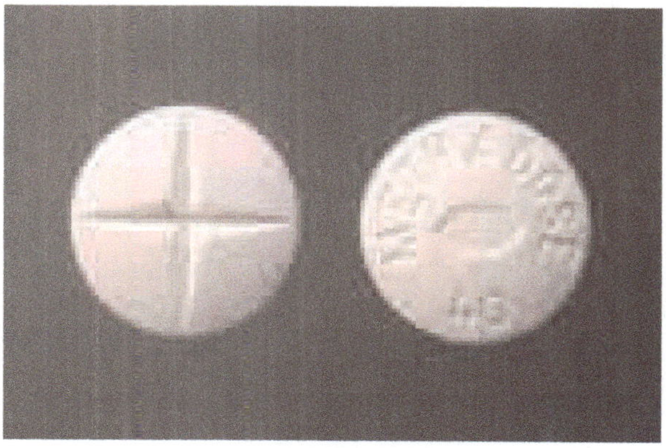

40 mg of methadone

Methadone maintenance treatment (MMT), a form of opioid replacement therapy, reduces and/or eliminates the use of illegal opiates, the criminality associated with opiate use, and allows patients to improve their health and social productivity. In addition, enrollment in methadone maintenance has the potential to reduce the transmission of infectious diseases associated with opiate injection, such as hepatitis and HIV. The principal effects of methadone maintenance are to relieve narcotic craving, suppress the abstinence syndrome, and block the euphoric effects associated with opiates. Methadone maintenance has been found to be medically safe and non-sedating. It is also indicated for pregnant women addicted to opiates. Methadone maintenance treatment is given to addicted individuals who feel unable to go the whole way and get clean. For individuals who wish to completely move away from drugs, they can start a methadone reduction program. A methadone reduction program is where an individual is prescribed an amount of methadone which is increased until withdrawal symptoms subside, after a period of stability, the dose will then be gradually reduced until the individual is either free of the need for methadone or is at a level which allows a switch to a different opiate with an easier withdrawal profile, such as Suboxone. Methadone toxicity has been shown to be associated with specific phenotypes of CYP2B6.

Some recovery in cognition are demonstrated after prolonged abstinence, but not in those using methadone.

Buprenorphine

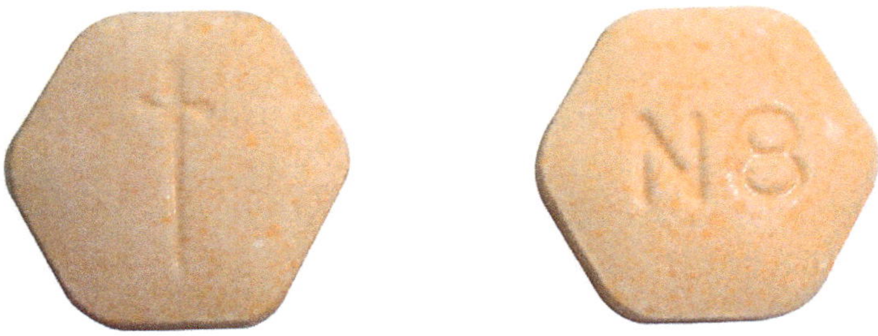

Suboxone tablet

Buprenorphine sublingual preparations are often used to manage opioid dependence (that is, dependence on heroin, oxycodone, hydrocodone, morphine, oxymorphone, fentanyl or other opioids). The Suboxone and Subutex preparations were approved for this indication by the United States Food and Drug Administration in October 2002. Some formulations of buprenorphine incorporate the opiate antagonist naloxone during the production of the pill form to prevent people from crushing the tablets and injecting them, instead of using the sublingual (under the tongue) route of administration.

Diamorphine

In Switzerland, Germany, the Netherlands, and the United Kingdom, long-term injecting drug users who do not benefit from methadone and other medication options are treated with pure injectable diamorphine that is administered under the supervision of medical staff. For this group of patients, diamorphine treatment has proven superior in improving their social and health situation.

Dihydrocodeine

Dihydrocodeine in both extended-release and immediate-release form are also sometimes used for maintenance treatment as an alternative to methadone or buprenorphine in some European countries.

Heroin-assisted Treatment

Heroin-assisted treatment (HAT, the medical prescription of heroin) has been available in Switzerland since 1994. A 2001 study found a high rate of treatment retention and significant improvement in health, social situation and likelihood to leave the illegal drug scene in enrolled participants. The study found that the most common reason for discharge was the start of abstinence treatment or methadone treatment. The study also found that heroin-assisted treatment is cost-beneficial on a society level due to reduced criminality and improved overall health of participants.

The heroin-assisted treatment program was introduced in Switzerland to combat the increase in heroin use in the 1980s and 1990s and written into law 2010 as one pillar of a four-pillar strategy using repression, prevention, treatment and risk reduction. Usually, only a small percentage of patients receives heroin and have to fulfil a number of criteria. Since then, HAT programs have been adopted in the Netherlands, United Kingdom, Germany, Spain, Denmark, Belgium, Canada, and Luxembourg.

Morphine (Extended-release)

An extended-release morphine confers a possible reduction of opioid use and with fewer depressive symptoms but overall more adverse effects when compared to other forms of long-acting opioids. Retention in treatment was not found to be significantly different. It is used in Switzerland.

Naltrexone

Naltrexone was approved by the FDA in 1984 for the treatment of opioid addiction by preventing relapse after detoxification (withdrawal). It is available both as an oral medication and as a monthly injectable (approved in 2010). Some authors question whether oral naltrexone is as effective in the treatment of opioid addiction as methadone and buprenorphine mainly due to non-compliance.

Behavioral Therapy

Twelve-step Programs

While medical treatment may help with the initial symptoms of opioid withdrawal, once an opiate addict overcomes the first stages of withdrawal, a method for long-term preventative care is attendance at 12-step groups such as Alcoholics Anonymous or Narcotics Anonymous. Attendance and participation in a 12-step program can be an effective way to obtain and maintain sobriety. Among primarily inner city minorities who had a "long severe history of (primarily) crack and/or heroin use", 51.7% of the individuals with continuous 12-step attendance had over 3 years of sustained abstinence, in contrast to 13.5% among those who had less than continuous 12-step attendance.

Epidemiology

Opioid use disorders resulted in 122,000 deaths worldwide in 2015, up from 18,000 deaths in 1990. Deaths from all causes rose from 47.5 million in 1990 to 55.8 million in 2013.

United States

In 2012 it was estimated that 9.2 percent of the population over the age of 12 years old had used an illicit drug in the previous month. In 2015, it was estimated the 20.5 million Americans had a substance use disorder. Of these 20.5 million, two million used prescribed pain medications (most of those being opioids) and one-half of a million were using heroin.

In 2015, in the US there were 33,000 deaths due to drug overdose that involved opioid use. Of these, about 15,000 were from prescribed opioids and 13,000 were from heroin use.

Non-medical consumption of opioids peaked around 2010 and then started to decrease between 2011 and 2013.

Among adults, the rate of inpatient hospital stays in the United States related to opioid overuse increased by an average of 5% annually from 1993–2012. The percentage of inpatient stays due to opioid overuse admitted from the emergency department increased from 43% in 1993 to 64% in 2005, but have remained relatively constant since 2005.

The prevalence of opioid use and opioid or opiate dependency varies by age and gender, among a myriad of other factors. Men are at higher risk for opioid use and dependency than women, and men also account for more opioid overdoses than women, although this gap is closing. Women are more likely to be prescribed pain relievers, be given higher doses, use them for longer durations, and may become dependent upon them faster.

Deaths due to opioid use also tend to skew at older ages than deaths from use of other illicit drugs. This does not reflect opioid use as a whole, which includes individuals in younger age demographics. Overdoses from opioids are highest among individuals who are between the ages of 40 and 50, in contrast to heroin overdoses, which are highest among individuals who are between the ages of 20 and 30. 21 to 35-year olds represent 77% of individuals who enter treatment for opioid use disorder, however, the average age of first-time use of prescription painkillers was 21.2 years of age in 2013.

History

Levacetylmethadol

Levacetylmethadol was previously used to treat opioid dependence. In 2003 the drug's manufacturer discontinued production. There are no available generic versions. LAAM produced long-lasting effects, which allowed the person receiving treatment to visit a clinic only three times per week, as opposed to daily as with methadone. In 2001, levacetylmethadol was removed from the European market due to reports of life-threatening ventricular rhythm disorders. In 2003, Roxane Laboratories, Inc. discontinued Orlaam in the US.

Amphetamine Dependence

Amphetamine dependence refers to a state of psychological dependence on a drug in the amphetamine class. In individuals with substance use disorder (problematic use or abuse with dependence), psychotherapy is currently the best treatment option as no pharmacological treatment has been approved. Tolerance is expected to develop with regular substituted amphetamine use. When substituted amphetamines are abused, drug tolerance develops rapidly.

Severe withdrawal associated with dependence from recreational substituted amphetamine use can be difficult for a user to cope with. Long-term use of certain substituted amphetamines, particularly methamphetamine, can reduce dopamine activity in the brain. Psychostimulants that increase dopamine and mimic the effects of substituted amphetamines, but with lower abuse liability, could theoretically be used as replacement therapy in amphetamine dependence. However, the few studies that used amphetamine, bupropion, methylphenidate and modafinil as a replacement therapy did not result in less methamphetamine use or craving.

In 2013, overdose on amphetamine, methamphetamine, and other compounds implicated in an "amphetamine use disorder" resulted in an estimated 3,788 deaths worldwide (3,425–4,145 deaths, 95% confidence).

References

- Pumariega A. J.; Rothe E.; Pumariega J. B. (2005). "Mental health of immigrants and refugees". Community Mental Health Journal. 41 (5): 581–597. doi:10.1007/s10597-005-6363-1
- (2002). Mosby's Medical, Nursing & Allied Health Dictionary. Sixth Edition. Drug abuse definition, p. 552. Nursing diagnoses, p. 2109. ISBN 0-323-01430-5
- Chambless, D.L.; et al. (1998). "An update on empirically validated therapies" (PDF). Clinical Psychology. American Psychological Association. 49: 5–14. Retrieved 2008-03-24
- Breitenfeld D.; Thaller V.; Perić B.; Jagetic N.; Hadžić D.; Breitenfeld T. (2008). "Substance abuse in performing musicians". Alcoholism: Journal on Alcoholism and Related Addictions. 44 (1): 37–42
- McCabe SE, Boyd CJ, Teter CJ (June 2009). "Subtypes of nonmedical prescription drug misuse". Drug Alcohol Depend. 102 (1–3): 63–70. PMC 2975029. PMID 19278795. doi:10.1016/j.drugalcdep.2009.01.007
- Evans, Katie; Sullivan, Michael J. (1 March 2001). Dual Diagnosis: Counseling the Mentally Ill Substance Abuser (2nd ed.). Guilford Press. pp. 75–76. ISBN 978-1-57230-446-8
- "Home Office | Tackling Drugs Changing Lives | Drugs in the workplace". 2007-06-09. Archived from the original on 2007-06-09. Retrieved 2016-09-19
- Longo, Dan L.; Schuckit, Marc A. (28 July 2016). "Treatment of Opioid-Use Disorders". New England Journal of Medicine. 375 (4): 357–368. doi:10.1056/NEJMra1604339
- Marc Galanter; Herbert D. Kleber (2008). The American Psychiatric Publishing textbook of substance abuse treatment. American Psychiatric Pub. p. 59. ISBN 978-1-58562-276-4. Retrieved 23 April 2010
- "What to do with leftover medicines". Medicines Talk, Winter 2005. Available at "Archived copy". Archived from the original on 2009-10-24. Retrieved 2010-01-06
- Lo CC, Cheng TC (2007). "The impact of childhood maltreatment on young adults' substance abuse". Am J Drug Alcohol Abuse. 33 (1): 139–46. PMID 17366254. doi:10.1080/00952990601091119
- Ruffle JK (Nov 2014). "Molecular neurobiology of addiction: what's all the (Δ)FosB about?". The American Journal of Drug and Alcohol Abuse. 40 (6): 428–37. PMID 25083822. doi:10.3109/00952990.2014.933840
- American Psychiatric Association (2013), Diagnostic and Statistical Manual of Mental Disorders (5th ed.), Arlington: American Psychiatric Publishing, pp. 540–546, ISBN 0890425558
- "Press Announcements - FDA approves first buprenorphine implant for treatment of opioid dependence". www.fda.gov. 26 May 2016. Retrieved 16 March 2017
- Joseph, H; Stancliff, S; Langrod, J (2000). "Methadone maintenance treatment (MMT): A review of historical and clinical issues". The Mount Sinai journal of medicine, New York. 67 (5–6): 347–64. PMID 11064485
- Sax KW, Strakowski SM (2001). "Behavioral sensitization in humans". J Addict Dis. 20 (3): 55–65. PMID 11681593. doi:10.1300/J069v20n03_06
- Substitution maintenance therapy in the management of opioid dependence and HIV/AIDS prevention (PDF). World Health Organization. 2004. ISBN 92-4-159115-3
- O'Connor, Patrick. "Amphetamines: Drug Use and Abuse". Merck Manual Home Health Handbook. Merck. Retrieved 26 September 2013

4

Understanding Addiction Psychology and Psychiatry

Addiction psychology consists of two parts, clinical and abnormal psychology. The two models of addicts considered by professional are diseases model of addiction and the choice model of addiction. Cognitive therapy and behaviorism are used to combat addiction. The chapter serves as a source to understand addiction psychology and psychiatry.

Addiction Psychology

Addiction psychology mostly comprises the clinical psychology and abnormal psychology disciplines and fosters the application of information obtained from research in an effort to appropriately diagnose, evaluate, treat, and support clients dealing with addiction. Throughout the treatment process addiction psychologists encourage behaviors that build wellness and emotional resilience to their physical, mental and emotional problems.

The basis of addiction is controversial. Professionals view it as a disease or a choice. One model is referred to as the Disease model of addiction. The second model is the Choice model of addiction. Researches argue that the addiction process is like the disease model with a target organ being the brain, some type of defect, and symptoms of the disease. The addiction is like the choice model with a disorder of genes, a reward, memory, stress, and choice. Both models result in compulsive behavior.

Cognitive Behavioral Therapy, Dialectal Behavior Therapy and Behaviorism are widely used approaches for addressing Process Addictions and Substance Addictions. Less common approaches are Eclectic, Psychodynamic, Humanistic, and Expressive therapies. Substance addictions are relate to drugs, alcohol, and smoking. Process addictions relate to non-substance related behaviors such as gambling, spending, sexual activity, gaming, internet, and food.

History

The word 'addiction' has successfully been traced to the 17th century. During this time period, addiction was defined as being compelled to act out any number of bad habits. Persons abusing narcotics were called opium and morphine 'eaters.' 'Drunkard' referred to abusers of alcohol. Medical textbooks categorized these 'bad habits' as dipsomania or alcoholism However, it wasn't until the 19th century when the diagnosis was first printed in medical literature. In the 1880s, Sigmund Freud and William Halsted began experimenting with users of cocaine. Unaware of the drug's powerful addictive qualities, they inadvertently became guinea pigs in their own research and, as a result, their contributions to psychology and medicine changed the world.

While working in Vienna General Hospital (Vienna Krankenhaus), in Austria, cocaine took possession over Freud's life when he found cocaine to relieve his migrane. When the effect of cocaine decreased, the amount of cocaine Freud consumed increased. With information about the pain suppressing properties of cocaine, physicians began prescribing cocaine to their patients who required pain relief.

Unaware of Freud and Halsted's experiments with cocaine, American Physician W.H. Bentley was conducting his own similar experiments. The Index Medicus published his article describing how he successfully treated patients with cocaine who were addicted to opium and alcohol. In the late 1800s the use of cocaine as a recreational drug spread like a worldwide epidemic.

As cocaine continued to spread physicians began looking for ways to treat patients with opium, cocaine, and alcohol addictions. Physicians debated the existence of the label 'addictive personality' but believed the qualities Freud possessed (bold risk taking, emotional scar tissue, and psychic turmoil) were of those that fostered the 'addictive personality'.

Important Contributors

Physician Sigmund Freud, born on May 6, 1856, in Freiberg, Moravia (an area now known as Pribor in the Czech Republic), was instrumental in the field of psychology. Dream interpretation and psychoanalysis (also known as talk therapy) are two of his well-known contributions. Psychoanalysis is used to treat a multitude of conditions including addictions.

William Halsted, born on September 23, 1852, in New York City, received his degree in medicine in 1877. Throughout his medical career as a surgeon he contributed surgical techniques that ultimately led to improvement of the patient's outcome following surgery. During Halsted's professional career, he (along with Freud) conducted experiments with the drug cocaine. While their research was in process they became guinea pigs for their own experiments when they became addicted to cocaine. In 1884 he became the first to describe how cocaine could be utilized as a localized anesthetic when injecting into the trunk of a sensory nerve, and how the localized ischemia prolonged the anesthetic properties of the drug.

G. Alan Marlatt was a pioneer in the field of addiction psychology. Born in Vancouver, British Columbia, in 1941, he spent his professional career as an addiction psychologist, researcher, and director of the University of Washington's Addictive Behaviors

Research Center and professor in the Department of Psychology. Marlatt adopted the theory of harm reduction, and developed and scientifically tested ways to prevent an addict's slip from becoming a relapse. He understood that expecting immediate and complete abstinence from addicts often deterred addicts from seeking the help they needed and deserved. Marlatt died on March 14, 2011.

A. Thomas McLellan was born in 1949 in Statan Island, New York. He is a professor at the University of Pennsylvania School of Medicine at the Center for Studies of Addiction. McLellan serves or has served on editorial boards as a reviewer of medical and scientific journals, and as an advisor to government and non-profit organizations including the National Practice Laboratory of the American Psychiatric Association, and the World Health Organization. He is co-founder and chief executive officer of the Treatment Research Institute located in Philadelphia, Pennsylvania. McLellan has conducted decades of research for the efficacy of treatment for substance abuse patients, and is recognized both at the national and international level as an addiction psychologist. He is also known for the development of the Addiction Severity Index or ASI and serves as editor-in-chief of the *Journal of Substance Abuse Treatment* and the deputy officer of National Drug Control Policy, Research and Evaluation.

Arnold Washton has specialized in addiction since 1975 and is a addiction psychologist known for his work in the development of therapeutic approaches to the treatment of drug and alcohol abuse. He is the author of many books and professional journal articles on treatment and addiction. He is a lecturer, clinician, researcher, and has served on the advisory committee for the US Food and Drug Administration. Washton is the founder and executive director of Recovery Options, a private addiction treatment practice located in New York City and Princeton, New Jersey.

William L. White is a Senior Research Consultant at Chestnut Health Systems, an addiction counselor, researcher and writer in the field of addiction for over 45 years. He wrote over 400 papers and 18 books. He received awards from the National Association of Addiction Treatment Providers (NAATP), the National Council on Alcoholism and Drug Dependence, (NAADAC), the Association of Addiction Professionals and the American Society of Addiction Medicine (ASAM).

Addiction

Addiction is a progressive disease and psychiatric disorder that is defined by the American Society of Addiction Medicine as "a primary, chronic disease of brain reward, motivation, memory and related circuitry. It is characterized by the inability to control behavior, it creates a dysfunctional emotional response, and it affects the users ability to abstain from the substance or behavior consistently. Psychology Today defines addiction as "a state that can occur when a person either consumes a substance such as nicotine, cocaine, or, alcohol or engages in an activity such as gambling or shopping/spending."

When a non-addict takes a drug or performs a behavior for the first time he/she does not automatically become an addict. Over time the non-addict chooses to continue to engage in a behavior or ingest a substance because of the pleasure the non-addict receives. The now addict has lost the ability to choose or forego the behavior or substance and the behavior becomes a compulsive action. The change from non-addict to addict occurs largely from the effects of prolonged substance use and behavior activities on brain functioning. Addiction affects the brain circuits of reward and motivation, learning and memory, and the inhibitory control over behavior.

There are different schools of thought regarding the terms dependence and addiction when referring to drugs and behaviors. One adopted belief is that "drug dependence" equals "addiction." The second belief is that the two terms do not equal each other. According to the DSM, the clinical criteria for "drug dependence" (or what we refer to as addiction) include compulsive drug use despite harmful consequences; inability to stop using a drug; failure to meet work, social, or family obligations; and, sometimes (depending on the drug), tolerance and withdrawal. The latter reflects physical dependence in which the body adapts to the drug, requiring more of it to achieve a certain effect (tolerance) and eliciting drug-specific physical or mental symptoms if drug use is abruptly ceased (withdrawal). Physical dependence can happen with the chronic use of many drugs—including even appropriate, medically instructed use. Thus, physical dependence in and of itself does not constitute addiction, but often accompanies addiction. This distinction can be difficult to discern, particularly with prescribed pain medications, where the need for increasing dosages can represent tolerance or a worsening underlying problem, as opposed to the beginning of abuse or addiction.

There are some characteristics of addiction that regardless of the type share commonalities. The behavior provides a rapid and potent means of altering mood, thoughts, and sensations of a person which occur because of physiology and learned expectations. The immediate precipitating factors of the relapse, the timing of the relapse and the rate of relapse following treatment is high.

American Psychological Association

The American Psychological Association (APA) is a professional psychological organization and is the largest association of psychologists in the United States. Over 100,000 researchers, educators, clinicians and students support the association through their membership. Their mission "is to advance the creation, communication and application of psychological knowledge to benefit society and improve people's lives."

APA supports 54 divisions, two of which pertain to addictions. Division 50, Society of Addiction Psychology promotes advances in research, professional training, and clinical practice within the range of addictive behaviors. Addictive behaviors include problematic use of alcohol, nicotine, and other drugs as well as disorders involving gambling, eating, spending, and sexual behavior. Division 28, Psychopharmacolgy and

Substance Abuse promotes teaching, research, and dissemination of information regarding the effects of drugs on behavior.

The College of Professional Psychology (CPP), hosted by the American Psychological Association Practice Organization, previously offered a certificate to psychologists whom demonstrated proficiency in the psychological treatment of alcohol and other substance-related disorders. The CPP maintains the certificate of proficiency for persons who acquired it prior to 2011. The Society of Addiction Psychology certificate will be re-instated while the Society examines other avenues for credentialing professionals in addiction treatment.

Addiction is not a "Disease"

40 years ago society was more judgmental towards people with addictions than they are now. Addicts were seen as abnormal and missing discipline and morality in their self-focused lives. When the idea of addiction being a disease was brought to life, people tended to not look so down on addicts. Addiction has very little in common with diseases. Addiction is behaviors and choices not an illness on its own. Addiction is self-acquired and is not transmissible, contagious, autoimmune, hereditary, degenerative, or traumatic. Diseases are illnesses, sicknesses, or ailments. Addiction is the symptom of the choice to use drugs and alcohol. Addiction is a choice, not a disease. Abstinence is the number one cure for addiction to drugs. There is no requirement for medical intervention to treat addiction, such as surgery.

Addiction as a Disease

It seems that wherever one finds intoxication, one likely will find addiction. Recently researchers have argued that the addiction process is like the disease model, with a target organ, a defect, and symptoms of the disease. In other accounts, addiction is a disorder of genes, reward, memory, stress, and choice.

The Disease Model in Addiction

According to the new disease model, rather than being a disease in the conventional sense, addiction is a disease of choice. That is, it is a disorder of the parts of the brain necessary to make proper decisions. As one becomes addicted to cocaine, the *ventral tegmentum nucleus accumbens* in the brain is the organ. The defect is stress-induced hedonic regulation.

Understanding the impact that genes, reward, memory, stress, and choice have on an individual will begin to explain the Disease Model of Addiction.

Genetic

The genetic makeup of an individual determines how they respond to alcohol. What causes an individual to be more prone to addiction is their genetic makeup. For example, there are genetic differences in how people respond to methylphenidate (Ritalin) injections.

Reward

Increased dopamine is correlated with increased pleasure. For that reason, dopamine plays a significant role in reinforcing experiences. It tells the brain the drug is better than expected. When an individual uses a drug, there may be a surge of dopamine in the midbrain, which can result in the shifting of that individual's pleasure "threshold" .

Memory

The neurochemical, glutamate is the most abundant neurochemical in the brain. It is critical in memory consolidation. When an addict discovers an addicting behavior, glutamate plays a role by creating the drug cues. It is the neurochemical in motivation which initiates the drug seeking, thus creating the addiction.

Stress

When under stress the brain is unable to achieve homeostasis. As a result, the brain reverts to allostasis, which in turn alters the brains ability to process pleasure, which is experienced at the hedonic "set point". Thus, previous pleasures may become no longer pleasurable. This is also known as anhedonia, or "pleasure deafness." When stressed, the addict may experience extreme craving—an intense, emotional, obsessive experience.

Choice

An addict may incur damage to the orbitofrontal cortex (OFC), the anterior cingulate cortex (ACC), and the prefrontal cortex (PFC). This damage causes a tendency to choose small and immediate rewards over larger but delayed rewards, deficits in social responding due to decreased awareness of social cues, and a failure of executive function such as sensitivity to consequences.

Addiction by Design

Addiction by Design describes the intensified forms of consumption that computer-based technologies enable and innovations deliberately enhance and sustain.

Licensed Practitioners

Many degrees provide space for the treatment of addictions. The educational background that each professional obtains will contain similarities but the philosophy and the viewpoint from which the material is delivered may vary. The required amount of education prior to earning a certificate or degree also varies. A few of the more commonly recognized fields of study are included.

- Psychologist
- Psychiatrist
- Licensed Counselor Social Worker
- Licensed Social Worker
- Licensed Professional Counselor
- Paraprofessional

Recognized Certifications in the Field of Addiction Psychology

Many certifications are recognized in the field of addiction psychology. Each have their own requirements.

- Certification for Alcohol and Drug Counselor Candidate.
- Credentialed Alcoholism and Substance Abuse Counselor.
- A Certified Chemical Dependency Counselor.
- Substance Abuse Counselor/Certified Addiction Counselor.
- The Certified Addiction Professional.
- Certified Addiction Treatment Counselors.
- Combined Certifications With Other Degrees.

Treatment

Both process addiction and behavioral addiction have many dimensions causing disarray in many aspects of the addicts' life. Treatment programs are not a one size fits all phenomenon, hence there are different modalities or levels of care. Effective treatment programs incorporate many components to address each dimension. The addict suffers from psychological dependence and some may suffer from physical dependence. Helping an individual stop using drugs is not enough. Addiction treatment must also help the individual maintain a drug-free lifestyle, and achieve productive functioning in the family, at work, and in society. Addiction is a disease which alters the structure and function of the brain. The brain circuitry may take months or years to recover after the addict has recovered. This may explain why drug abusers are at risk for relapse even after long periods of abstinence and despite the potentially devastating consequences. Research shows that most addicted individuals need a minimum of 3 months in treatment to significantly reduce or stop their drug use, however treatment in excess of 3 months has a greater success rate. Recovery from addiction is a longterm process.

Modalities of Care

The modality or level of care needed for a patient is decided by the treating professional in conjunction with the patient when feasible. As expected the patient receiving treatment will likely take steps forward and backward the level of care will likely to fluctuate. Common modalities are explained.

Detoxification and Medically Managed Withdrawal

The process when the body rids itself of drugs is referred to as detoxification, and is usually concurrent with the side effects of withdrawal which vary depending on the substance(s) and are often unpleasant and even fatal. Physicians may prescribe a medication that will help decrease the withdrawal symptoms while the addict is receiving care in an inpatient or outpatient setting. Detoxification is generally considered a precursor to or a first stage of treatment because it is designed to manage the acute and potentially dangerous physiological effects of stopping drug use.

Long-term Residential

Treatment is structured and operates 24 hours a day. Residents will remain in treatment from usually 6 to 12 months while developing accountability, responsibility and socialization skills. Activities are designed to help addicts recover from destructive behavior patterns while adopting positive behavioral patterns. Constructive methods of interacting with others and improving self-esteem are other areas of focus. The therapeutic community model is an example of one treatment approach. Many therapeutic communities provide a more comprehensive approach to include employment training and other support services.

Short-term Residential

Short-term residential programs are on average 3–6 weeks in a residential setting. The program is intensive followed by more extended outpatient treatment to include individual and/or group therapy, 12-step Anonymous programs, or other forms of support. Because of the short duration of this modality it is even more important for individuals to remain active in outpatient treatment programs to help decrease the risk of relapse following residential treatment.

Outpatient-treatment Programs

Outpatient treatment program vary regarding the services offered and the intensity. It's more affordable and may be more suitable for patients who are employed full-time and/or who have secured multiple social supports. Outpatient programs may include group and/or individual therapy, intensive outpatient program, and partial hospitalization. Some outpatient programs are also designed to treat patients with medical or other mental health problems in addition to their drug disorders.

Individualized Drug Counseling

Individualized drug counseling not only focuses on reducing or stopping illicit drug or alcohol use; it also addresses related areas of impaired functioning such as employment status, illegal activity, and family/social relations as well as the content and structure of the patient's recovery program. Through its emphasis on short-term behavioral goals, individualized counseling helps the patient develop coping strategies and tools to abstain from drug use and maintain abstinence. The addiction counselor encourages 12-step participation (at least one or two times per week) and makes referrals for needed supplemental medical, psychiatric, employment, and other services.

Group Counseling

An outpatient treatment option facilitated by a treatment provider and used to expand on the support system the patient already has. Groups foster a non-judgmental environment allowing patients to meet and discuss difficulties and successes of their addiction while providing on-going support that is needed to be successful with recovery.

Intensive Outpatient Program (IOP)

As the name implies this is an outpatient treatment option designed for addicts who for various reasons do not have the opportunity to attend an inpatient treatment program, yet who otherwise would not be able to receive the level of support needed to recover from their addiction. Programs vary in duration based on the patients need. Because of the lower level of support offered IOP is frequently used as a step down approach from patients leaving inpatient treatment but who are still in need of intensive therapy.

Prevention, Relapse & Recovery

Therapeutic Orientations & Approaches

In 1878 the Index Medicus published research conducted and written by American physician W.H. Bentley. Bentley's research described his success in treating patients addicted to the 'opium habit' w/cocaine. Two years later he reported success in treating both opium and alcohol abusers w/cocaine. Today, the swapping one addiction for another is referred to as crossover addiction.

A variety of treatment approaches are utilized by health professionals in order to provide their clients the highest possible level of success to overcome their addictions. There is no one specific approach and often therapists will use multiple techniques.

- Behaviorism.
- Humanistic Therapy.

- Cognitive Behavioral Therapy (CBT).
- Dialectical Behavioral Therapy (DBT).
- Psychodynamic.
- Expressive.
- Integrative.
- Harm Reduction.
- Eclectic.
- Animal Assisted Therapy.

Addiction Vulnerability

Addiction vulnerability is the genetic, physiological, or psychological predisposition to engage in addictive behaviors. A vulnerability to addiction may lead to an increased risk for a substance dependence. Addictions can arise in both a chemical and a behavioral manner. A chemical addiction refers to a physical substance dependence where a behavioral addiction involves a psychological dependence. Genetics has been shown to account for 40–60% of a person's likelihood to develop an addiction. Research is working toward establishing a comprehensive picture of the neurobiology of addiction vulnerability, including all factors at work in propensity for addiction.

Substance Addiction

A physical, chemical addiction refers to the repeated and uncontrollable abuse of drugs or alcohol. To be physically addicted to a substance means that the normal release of neurotransmitter has been obstructed by the presence of a chemical of abuse. The reward center of the brain gets overstimulated with the pleasurable response of drug or alcohol use and adapts to accommodate these increase levels of chemical input. This creates a neural environment for addiction development. Natural neural reuptake receptors become desensitized to the drug due to repeated exposure and have to adapt to function properly only in the presence of compounding amounts of the substance.

According to the American Psychiatric Association, substance use disorder is a complex behavioral disorder characterized by compulsive drug use, the development of tolerance and withdrawal, and overall functional impairment. In the Diagnostic and Statistical Manual of Mental Disorders IV-TR (DSM-IV-TR) substance use disorder was split into two categories: abuse and dependence. The American Psychiatric Association lists the criteria for the potentiality of drug abuse. Those criteria are: (a) recurrent failure to fulfill major role obligations; (b) recurrent use of the substance in situations in which it might be hazardous; (c) recurrent substance-related legal problems; and (d) continued substance use despite having persistent or recurrent social or interpersonal problems. A substance dependence diagnosis was met if three or more of the following criteria were fulfilled: (a) tolerance; (b) withdrawal; (c) using larger amounts or over a longer period of time than intended; (d) a persistent desire or unsuccessful efforts to cut down or control use; (e) spending a great deal of time obtaining, (f) using or recovering from the effects of the substance; (g) reducing or giving up important activities due to substance use; and (h) persistent physical or psychological problem that are likely due to or exacerbated by the substance.

With the revised edition of the Diagnostic and Statistical Manual of Mental Disorders (DSM-5) there has been a shift from the traditional categorization of addiction as substance abuse and/or dependence to a more dimensional model that combines the diagnostic criteria from both "abuse" and "dependence" into a singular disorder. The criteria for diagnosis remains relatively the same in the DSM-5 with a few changes such as the removal of "recurrent legal problems" criteria, the addition of "craving or a strong desire to use the substance," and the threshold for diagnosis has been revised to include positive identification with two or more criteria. The shift from a categorical to a more dimensional approach exemplifies the evolving conceptualization of addiction in the field.

Three-factor Model

Accepted research now shows that some people have vulnerabilities to addiction and has established a three-factor standard for vulnerability to drug addiction: genetic factors, environmental factors and repeated exposure to drugs of abuse. Being vulnerable to addiction means that there exists some factor which makes one individual more likely to develop an addiction than another individual. Additionally, many in the science community agree that addiction is not simply just a result of desensitized neural receptors but also a corollary of long-term associated memories (or cues) of substance use and self-administration. Vulnerability to addiction has both physiological and psychological components.

Genetic Factors

Contemporary research in the neurobiology of addiction points to genetics as a major contributing factor to addiction vulnerability. It has been estimated that 40–60% of the vulnerability to developing an addiction is due to genetics. One gene in particular, the D_2 subtype of dopamine receptor, has been studied at length in association to substance addiction. The D_2 receptor responds to the chemical dopamine which produces rewarding and pleasurable feelings in the brain. Through mice studies, agreeing contemporary research has shown that individuals with a deficiency in this dopamine receptor exhibit not only a preference for and increased consumption of alcohol over their genetically normal peers, but also compensated levels of the cannabinoid receptor type CB_1. This suggests that both of these genetic factors work together in the regulation of alcohol and cocaine in the brain and in the normal regulation of dopamine. Individuals with this genetic deficiency in the D_2 dopamine receptor may be more likely to seek out these recreational pleasure/reward producing substances as they are less receptive to the natural "feel good" effects of dopamine. This naturally occurring deficiency is one of the most studied genetic vulnerabilities to substance abuse across the field. Recent studies show that GABA also plays a role in vulnerability to addiction. When alcohol is consumed it affects GABA by mimicking its effects on the brain, such as basic motor functions.

Additionally, genetics play a role on individual traits, which may put one at increased risk for experimentation with drugs, continued use of drugs, addictions, and potential for relapse. Some of these individual personality traits, such as impulsivity, reward-seeking, and response to stress, may lead to increased vulnerability to addiction.

Environmental Factors

A major environmental factor that increases vulnerability to developing addiction is availability of drugs. Additionally, other environmental factors come into play, such as socioeconomic status and poor familial relationships, and have been shown to be contributing factors in the initiation (and continued use) of drug abuse. Neurobiology again plays a role in addiction vulnerability when in combination with environmental factors. The main risk of chronic stressors contributing to vulnerability is that they can put the brain in a compromised state. External stressors (such as financial concerns and family problems) can, after repeated exposure, affect the physiology of the brain. Chronic stress or trauma has been shown to have neuroadaptive effects such that the brain can essentially physically "rewire" itself to accommodate for the increase in cortisol produced by the stressors. Evidence has also shown that a great amount of stress hinders your prefrontal functioning as well causes an increased limbic-stratal level responding. This can lead to low behavioral and cognitive control. Additionally, when the brain is put under severe stress due to repeated drug use, it has been shown to be physiologically altered. This compromised neural state plays a large role in perpetuating addiction and in making recovery more difficult.

Adolescence

Previous research has examined the increased risk of substance use initiation during adolescence. Many factors have been identified as being associated with increased risk of substance use during this period of development including individual differences (e.g., negative affect, decreased harm avoidance, and low motivation for achievement), biological (e.g., genetic predisposition and neurological development), and environmental factors (e.g., high levels of stress, peer influences, availability of substances, etc.) Rat studies provide behavioral evidence that adolescence is a period of increased vulnerability to drug-seeking behavior and onset addiction. The mesolimbic dopamine system of the brain is undergoing reorganization and functional changes during adolescence. Rat studies have demonstrated that adolescents have tendencies and abilities to drink more than adults due to minimal disruption to their motor functions and also due to minimal sensitivity to sedation. As a result, it is more susceptible to become addicted in the wake of drug use during this developmental period. Overall, social, behavioral and developmental factors in adolescence make individuals more liable to drug seeking behavior, and as a result, addiction.

Repeated Exposure

Repeated exposure to a drug is one of the determining factors in distinguishing recreational substance use from chronic abuse. Many neurobiological theories of addiction place repeated or continued use of the drug in the path of addiction development. For example, researchers have theorized that addiction is the result of the shift from goal-directed actions to habits and ultimately, to compulsive drug-seeking and taking. In other words, repeated, deliberate use of the drug plays a role in the eventual compulsory drug-taking and/or habitual drug-taking associated with addiction. Another theory suggests that through repeated use of the drug, individuals become sensitized to drug-associated stimuli which may result in compulsive motivation and desire for the drug. Additionally, a third neurobiological theory highlights the changes in brain reward circuitry following repeated drug use that contributes to the development of addiction such that addiction is conceptualized as being a progression of allostatic changes in which the addicted individual is able to maintain stability but at a pathological set point. Experience-dependent neural plasticity is a hallmark of repeated drug exposure and refers to the adaptation of the brain due to increased levels of the drug in the body. In this sense, repeated exposure falls under the both physiological vulnerability and behavioral/psychological vulnerability to addiction.

Although many variables individually contribute to an increased risk of developing a substance use disorder, no single vulnerability guarantees the development of addiction. It is the combination of many factors (e.g. genetics, environmental stressors, initiation and continued use of the drug) that culminates in the development of this disorder.

Addiction Psychiatry

Addiction psychiatry founded in 1991, is a medical subspecialty within psychiatry that focuses on the evaluation, diagnosis, and treatment of people who are suffering from one or more disorders related to addiction. This may include disorders involving legal and illegal drugs, gambling, sex, food, and other impulse control disorders. Addiction psychiatrists are substance abuse experts. Growing amounts of scientific knowledge, such as the health effects and treatments to substance abuse, have led to advancements in the field of addiction psychiatry. These advancements in understanding the neurobiology of rewarding behavior, along with federal funding, has allowed for ample opportunity for research in the discipline of addiction psychiatry. Addiction psychiatry is an expanding field, and currently there is a high demand for substance abuse experts in both the private and public sector.

History

Addicition psychiatry is a relatively new subspecialty of psychiatry. As of October 1991, the American Board of Psychiatry and Neurology and the American Board of Medical Specialties (ABMS), with support of the American Psychiatric Association, established a "Committee on Certification of Added Qualifications in Addiction Psychiatry." This was a way to identify the most educated and experienced psychiatrists in the profession; however, it was not until 1993 when "Addiction Psychiatry" was granted sub-specialization status. Years later, in 1997 the committee's board of trustees along with the ABMS renamed the committee "Committee on Certification in the Subspecialty of Addiction Psychiatry". The committee became more geared toward developing the subspecialty of addiction psychiatry. As of 1997, there were only 13 addiction psychiatry programs that the Accreditation Council for Graduate Medical Education(ACGME) recognized. Currently the ACGME recognizes 45 different residency programs in the United States.

Profession

Qualifications

In order to become a certified addiction psychiatrist one must first have completed medical school and further be certified as a general psychiatrist. Next, general psychiatrists must commit themselves to an ACGME-accredited residency in addiction psychiatry. The addiction psychiatry residencies are one-year programs set in a hospital or clinical setting where general psychiatrists learn how to diagnose and treat substance-use disorders as well as potential coexisting psychiatric disorders. After completing one of these residency programs addiction psychiatrists are then capable of being hired in either a private or public setting.

Status

An increase in pressure from local and federal governments to provide for patients suffering from addiction has resulted in the increased demand for addiction psychiatrists. Federal funding for the prevention of addiction has been carried out via block grants. These investments in addiction treatment yield savings in overall societal costs, as general health care costs diminish. As of October 2010, the average salary of addiction psychiatrists was $151,000. Additionally, 47 addiction psychiatrist appeared on US News and World Report's list of US News Top Doctors. A further 16 addiction psychiatrists were nominated by their peers to an even more selective group of America's Top Doctors.

Treatment

Background

Addiction psychiatry aims to treat individuals with addiction issues along with co-occurring psychiatric disorders, otherwise known as patients with dual diagnosis. Addiction psychiatrists treat a wide variety of patients of all ages with varying conditions. Each case of addiction is unique and addiction psychiatrists must cater to each individual patient. Addiction psychiatrists must recognize the numerous factors that tie into each individual's struggle with an addiction. For example, substance abuse often occurs among individuals dealing with mood disorders and other social stresses. Addiction psychiatrists must be able to recognize, diagnose, and treat the disorders concurrent with the substance abuse issues. Furthermore, addiction psychiatrists must also recognize certain health effects from illicit drugs in order to properly treat each individual.

Methodology

Addiction psychiatry encompasses both medicine and psychotherapy, or professional therapeutic interaction, as the means of treating individuals. However, not all substance addictions contain approved medication for treatment. In a conventional addiction psychiatry session, addiction psychiatrists will gain a better understanding of their patient's lifestyle by gathering medical history and the patient's mental health concerns. Next, the psychiatrist will construct different possible solutions to the patient's problem; if necessary addiction psychiatrists will prescribe medication. Moreover, addiction psychiatrists recommend the benefits of 12-Step programs such as Narcotics Anonymous and Alcoholics Anonymous and often encourage patients to seek external support. Addiction psychiatry can also be a method of recovery for those who have attempted to cease their drug or alcohol abuse without prior success.

References

- Mayfield, R. D.; Harris, R. A.; Schuckit, M. A. (2008). "Genetic factors influencing alcohol dependence". British Journal of Pharmacology. 154 (2): 275–287. doi:10.1038/bjp.2008.88
- American Psychological Association. "American Psychological Association". American Psychological Association. Retrieved 15 September 2012
- Olch, Peter D. (March 2006). "William Stewart Halsted". Annals of Surgery. Lippincott, Williams, and Wilkins. 243 (3): 418–25. PMC 1448951. PMID 16495709. doi:10.1097/01.sla.0000201546.94163.00
- Beck, Judith (2011). Cognitive Behavioral Therapy: Basics and Beyond (second ed.). New York: Guilford Press. pp. 2–10. ISBN 978-1609185046

- Kalivas, P. W., & Volkow, N. D. (2005). The neural basis of addiction: A Pathology of Motivation and Choice. The American Journal Of Psychiatry,162(8), 1403-1413
- Behavioral Medicine Associates. "The Addictive Process". Psychiatry and Wellness:Behavioral Medicine Associates. Retrieved 24 October 2012
- Holden T (2012). "Addiction is not a disease". CMAJ. 184: 679. PMC 3314045. PMID 22473931. doi:10.1503/cmaj.112-2033
- Watson, John B. (1998). Behaviorism (7th printing ed.). New Brunswick, NJ: Transaction Publishers. pp. 11, 16. ISBN 978-1-56000-994-8
- Marlatt, Alan G. (November–December 1996). "Harm reduction: come as you are". Journal of Addictive Behaviors. 21 (6): 779–88. ISSN 0306-4603. PMID 8904943. doi:10.1016/0306-4603(96)00042-1
- American Academy of Addiction Psychiatry, "Trainee FAQ", 2012, ""Archived copy". Archived from the original on 2013-02-18. Retrieved 2013-02-16. ", 2/2/13
- Hiroi, Agatsuma (2005). "Genetic susceptibility to substance dependence". Mol Psychiatry. 10 (4): 336–44. PMID 15583701. doi:10.1038/sj.mp.4001622
- Lewis, Marc (2015). The Biology of Desire: Why Addiction is not a disease. New York: Public Affairs. ISBN 978-1-61039-437-6
- John T. Pichot, MD, Luz Starck, MD, John T. Harris, MD, Jeffrey M. Benzick, MD, Medscape Psychiatry & Mental Health eJournal, "Addiction Psychiatry: Training, Certification, and Internet Resources", 1997, "[6]"
- "International Expressive Arts Therapy Association". International Expressive Arts Therapy Association. Archived from the original on 7 June 2012. Retrieved 30 September 2012
- Koob, G. F. (2003). "Alcoholism: Allostasis and Beyond". Alcoholism: Clinical and Experimental Research. 27 (2): 232–243. doi:10.1097/01.ALC.0000057122.36127

5

Treatment for Addiction

Addiction can be treated by therapy, counseling or by medication. Addiction medicine is the treatment given for addiction. Drug rehabilitation, nicotine replacement therapy, coding, contingency management and community reinforcement approach and family training are some diagnosis and treatments discussed in the following section. Addiction is best understood in confluence with the major topics listed in the following chapter.

Addiction Medicine

Addiction medicine is a medical specialty that deals with the treatment of addiction. The specialty often crosses over into other areas, since various aspects of addiction fall within the fields of public health, psychology, social work, mental health counseling, psychiatry, and internal medicine, among others. Incorporated within the specialty are the processes of detoxification, rehabilitation, harm reduction, abstinence-based treatment, individual and group therapies, oversight of halfway houses, treatment of withdrawal-related symptoms, acute intervention, and long term therapies designed to reduce likelihood of relapse. Some specialists, primarily those who also have expertise in family medicine or internal medicine, also provide treatment for disease states commonly associated with substance use, such as hepatitis and HIV infection.

Physicians specializing in the field are in general agreement concerning applicability of treatment to those with addiction to drugs, such as alcohol and heroin, and often also to gambling, which has similar characteristics and has been well-described in the scientific literature. There is less agreement concerning definition or treatment of other so-called addictive behavior such as sexual addiction and internet addiction, such behaviors not being marked generally by physiologic tolerance or withdrawal.

Doctors focusing on addiction medicine are medical specialists who focus on addictive disease and have had special study and training focusing on the prevention and treatment of such diseases. There are two routes to specialization in the addiction field: one via a psychiatric pathway and one via other fields of medicine. The American Society of Addiction Medicine notes that approximately 40% of its members are psychiatrists (MD/DO) while the remainder have received primary medical training in other fields.

In several countries around the world, specialist bodies have been set up to ensure high quality practice in addiction medicine. For example, within the United States, there are two accepted specialty examinations. One is a Board Certification in Addiction Psychiatry from the American Board of Psychiatry and Neurology. The other is a Board Certification in Addiction Medicine from the American Board of Preventive Medicine. The latter approach is available to all physicians with primary Board certification, while the former is available only to board-certified psychiatrists. Doctors of Osteopathic Medicine may also seek board certification via the American Osteopathic Association (AOA). The Doctor of Osteopathic Medicine must have a primary board certification in Neurology & Psychiatry or Internal Medicine from the American Osteopathic Association and complete an AOA approved addiction medicine fellowship. Successful completion of a board examination administered via the AOA will grant a certificate of added qualification (CAQ) in addiction medicine.

Within Australia, addiction medicine specialists are certified via the Chapter of Addiction Medicine, which is part of the Royal Australasian College of Physicians. They may alternatively be a member of the Section of Addiction Psychiatry, Royal Australian & New Zealand College of Psychiatrists.

The International Society of Addiction Medicine also can provide certification of expertise.

Acamprosate

Acamprosate, sold under the brand name Campral, is a medication used along with counselling to treat alcohol dependence.

Acamprosate is thought to stabilize the chemical balance in the brain that would otherwise be disrupted by alcohol withdrawal. Studies find that acamprosate works to best advantage in combination with psychosocial support and can help facilitate reduced consumption as well as full abstinence.

Serious side effects include allergic reactions, abnormal heart rhythms, and low or high blood pressure, while less serious side effects include headaches, insomnia, and impotence. Diarrhea is the most common side-effect. Acamprosate should not be taken by people with kidney problems or allergies to the drug.

Until it became a generic in the United States, Campral was manufactured and marketed in the United States by Forest Laboratories, while Merck KGaA markets it outside the US. It is sold as 333 mg white and odorless tablets of acamprosate calcium, which is the equivalent of 300 mg of acamprosate.

Medical Uses

Acamprosate is useful when used along with counselling in the treatment of alcohol dependence. Over three to twelve months it increases the number of people who do not drink at all and the number of days without alcohol. It appears to work as well as naltrexone.

Contraindications

Acamprosate is primarily removed by the kidneys and should not be given to people with severely impaired kidneys (creatinine clearance less than 30ml/min). A dose reduction is suggested in those with moderately impaired kidneys (creatinine clearance between 30ml/min and 50ml/min). It is also contraindicated in those who have a strong allergic reaction to acamprosate calcium or any of its components.

Interactions

Current studies have not shown any serious drug-drug interactions between acamprosate and alcohol, diazepam, imipramine, or disulfiram. One study found that giving acamprosate with naltrexone had no harmful effects and no clinically important effects on the pharmacokinetics of either drugs.

Pharmacology

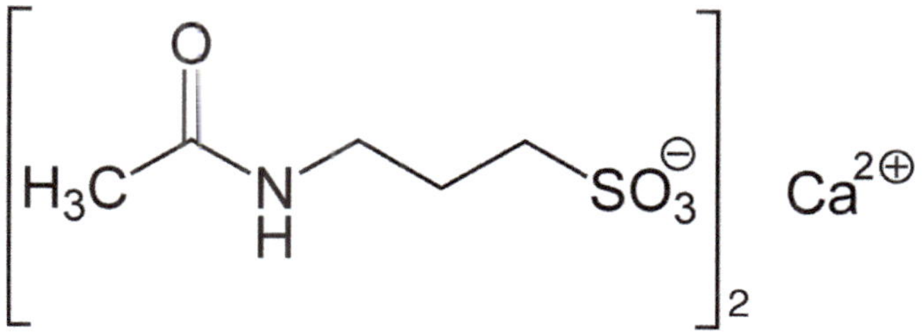

acamprosate calcium

The mechanism of action of acamprosate is unknown and controversial. At high concentrations, well above those that occur clinically (1–3 μM), reports of inhibition of glutamate receptor-activated responses (1 mM), enhancement of NMDA receptor function (300 μM), weak antagonization of the NMDA receptor, partial agonism of the polyamine site of the NMDA receptor, and possible inhibition of the mGluR1 and mGluR5 (10 μM) have all been published. However, no direct action of acamprosate at clinically-relevant concentrations has yet been reported. Moreover, a subsequent study found no action of acamprosate on the mGluR1 or mGluR5 at concentrations as high as 100 μM, nor at $GABA_A$ or glycine receptors or voltage-gated sodium channels.

GABA

Ethanol and benzodiazepines act on the central nervous system by binding to the $GABA_A$ receptor, increasing the effects of the inhibitory neurotransmitter GABA (i.e., it is a positive allosteric modulator). In chronic alcohol abuse, one of the main mechanisms of tolerance is attributed to $GABA_A$ receptors becoming downregulated (i.e. becoming generally less sensitive to the inhibitory effect of the GABA system). When alcohol is no longer consumed, these down-regulated $GABA_A$ receptor complexes are so insensitive to GABA that the typical amount of GABA produced has little effect; compounded with the fact that GABA normally inhibits action potential formation, there are not as many receptors for GABA to bind to – meaning that sympathetic activation is unopposed, leading to sympathetic over-stimulation. Acamprosate's mechanism of action is supposed to be, at least partially, due to an enhancement effect on GABA receptors. It has been purported to open the chloride ion channel in a novel way as it does not require GABA as a cofactor, making it less liable for dependence than benzodiazepines. Acamprosate has been successfully used to control tinnitus, hyperacusis, ear pain and inner ear pressure during alcohol use due to spasms of the tensor tympani muscle.

NMDA

In addition, alcohol also inhibits the activity of *N*-methyl-D-aspartate receptors (NMDARs). Chronic alcohol consumption leads to the overproduction (upregulation) of these receptors. Thereafter, sudden alcohol abstinence causes the excessive numbers of NMDARs to be more active than normal and to contribute to the symptoms of delirium tremens and excitotoxic neuronal death. Withdrawal from alcohol induces a surge in release of excitatory neurotransmitters like glutamate, which activates NMDARs. Acamprosate reduces this glutamate surge. The drug also protects cultured cells from excitotoxicity induced by ethanol withdrawal and from glutamate exposure combined with ethanol withdrawal.

Calcium

In contrast to the aforementioned wide array of purported mechanisms of action, a 2013 profile animal study published in *Neuropsychopharmacology* suggests that acamprosate has by itself no psychotropic profile, no *N*-methyl-D-aspartate receptor or metabotropic glutamate receptor 5 activity, and that therapeutic effects are due to the active calcium moiety co-administered with the acamprosate salt form. These findings have not yet been reproduced.

Neuroprotective Effects

In addition to its apparent ability to help patients refrain from drinking, some evidence suggests that acamprosate is neuroprotective (that is, it protects neurons from damage and death caused by the effects of alcohol withdrawal, and possibly other causes of neurotoxicity). For example, acamprosate has been found to protect cultured cells from damage induced by ischemia (inadequate blood flow). The drug also protected infant hamsters from brain damage induced by injections of the toxin ibotenic acid (which exacerbates excitotoxicity, the harmful over-activation of glutamate receptors).

One Brazilian study has shown that acamprosate may be an effective treatment for tinnitus.

Society and Culture

Names

"Acamprosate" is the INN and BAN for this substance. "Acamprosate calcium" is the USAN and JAN. It is also technically known as *N*-acetylhomotaurine or as calcium acetylhomotaurinate.

It is sold under the brand name Campral.

Approval

While the Food and Drug Administration (FDA) in the United States approved this drug in July 2004, it has been legal in Europe since 1989. After it approved the drug, the FDA released this statement:

While its mechanism of action is not fully understood, Campral is thought to act on the brain pathways related to alcohol abuse. Campral was demonstrated to be safe and effective by multiple placebo-controlled clinical studies involving alcohol-dependent patients who had already been withdrawn from alcohol, (i.e., detoxified). Campral proved superior to placebo in maintaining abstinence (keeping patients off alcohol consumption), as indicated by a greater percentage of acamprosate-treated subjects being assessed as continuously abstinent throughout treatment. Campral is not addicting and was generally well tolerated in clinical trials. The most common adverse events reported for patients taking Campral included headache, diarrhea, flatulence, and nausea.

Disulfiram

Disulfiram (sold under the trade names Antabuse and Antabus) is a drug discovered in the 1920s used to support the treatment of chronic alcoholism by producing an acute sensitivity to ethanol (drinking alcohol). Disulfiram works by inhibiting the enzyme acetaldehyde dehydrogenase, which means that many of the effects of a "hangover" are felt immediately after alcohol is consumed. "Disulfiram plus alcohol, even small amounts, produce flushing, throbbing in head and neck, throbbing headache, respiratory difficulty, nausea, copious vomiting, sweating, thirst, chest pain, palpitation, dyspnea, hyperventilation, tachycardia, hypotension, syncope, marked uneasiness, weakness, vertigo, blurred vision, and confusion. In severe reactions there may be respiratory depression, cardiovascular collapse, arrhythmias, myocardial infarction, acute congestive heart failure, unconsciousness, convulsions, and death"

In the body, alcohol is converted to acetaldehyde, which is then broken down by acetaldehyde dehydrogenase. If the dehydrogenase enzyme is inhibited, acetaldehyde builds up and causes unpleasant effects. Disulfiram should be used in conjunction with counseling and support.

Disulfiram is also being studied as a treatment for cocaine dependence, as it prevents the breakdown of dopamine (a neurotransmitter whose release is stimulated by cocaine); the excess dopamine results in increased anxiety, elevated blood pressure, restlessness, and other unpleasant symptoms. Several studies have reported that it has antiprotozoal activity, as well. Disulfiram is the subject of research for treatment of cancer and HIV (to activate the reservoir of HIV-infected resting CD4 cells).

Uses

Alcoholism

Under normal metabolism, alcohol is broken down in the liver by the enzyme alcohol dehydrogenase to acetaldehyde, which is then converted by the enzyme acetaldehyde dehydrogenase to a harmless acetic acid derivative (acetyl coenzyme A). Disulfiram blocks this reaction at the intermediate stage by blocking acetaldehyde dehydrogenase. After alcohol intake under the influence of disulfiram, the concentration of acetaldehyde in the blood may be five to 10 times higher than that found during metabolism of the same amount of alcohol alone. As acetaldehyde is one of the major causes of the symptoms of a "hangover", this produces immediate and severe negative reaction to alcohol intake. Some five to 10 minutes after alcohol intake, the patient may experience the effects of a severe hangover for a period of 30 minutes up to several hours. Symptoms include flushing of the skin, accelerated heart rate, shortness of breath, nausea, vomiting, throbbing headache, visual disturbance, mental confusion, postural syncope, and circulatory collapse.

Disulfiram should not be taken if alcohol has been consumed in the last 12 hours. There is no tolerance to disulfiram: the longer it is taken, the stronger its effects. As disulfiram is absorbed slowly through the digestive tract and eliminated slowly by the body, the effects may last for up to two weeks after the initial intake; consequently, medical ethics dictate that patients must be fully informed about the disulfiram-alcohol reaction.

A nine-year study published in 2006 found that incorporation of supervised disulfiram and a related compound calcium carbimide into a comprehensive treatment program resulted in an abstinence rate of over 50%.

Disulfiram does not reduce alcohol cravings, so a major problem associated with this drug is extremely poor compliance. A classic study by Fuller (1986) that followed chronic alcoholics for a period of one year found no statistically significant differences in abstinence rates between the group that received disulfiram and the group that only received counseling. The reason for this finding was that only 20% of subjects in disulfiram group were estimated to be in good compliance with the drug regimen. Methods to improve compliance include subdermal implants, which release the drug continuously over a period of up to 12 weeks, and supervised administration practices, for example, having the drug regularly administered by one's spouse.

Although disulfiram remained the most common pharmaceutical treatment of alcohol abuse till the end of the 20th century, today it is often replaced or accompanied with newer drugs, primarily the combination of naltrexone and acamprosate, which directly attempt to address physiological processes in the brain associated with alcohol abuse.

Cancer

When disulfiram creates complexes with metals (dithiocarbamate complexes), it is a proteasome inhibitor and can represent a new approach to proteasome inhibition. Clinical trials are recommended. A clinical trial of disulfiram with copper gluconate against liver cancer is being conducted in Utah (ClinicalTrials.gov Identifier: NCT00742911) and a clinical trial of disulfiram as adjuvant against lung cancer is happening in Israel (ClinicalTrials.gov Identifier: NCT00312819).

Side Effects in Absence of Alcohol

The most common side effects in the absence of alcohol are headache, and a metallic or garlic taste in the mouth, though more severe side effects may occur. Tryptophol, a chemical compound that induces sleep in humans, is formed in the liver after disulfiram treatment. Less common side effects include decrease in libido, liver problems, skin rash, and nerve inflammation.

Cases of disulfiram neurotoxicity have also occurred, causing extrapyramidal and other symptoms.

Disulfiram disrupts metabolism of several other compounds, including paracetamol (acetaminophen), theophylline and caffeine. However, in most cases, this disruption is mild and presents itself as a 20–40% increase in the half-life of the compound at typical dosages of disulfiram.

Similarly Acting Substances

In medicine, the term "disulfiram effect" refers to an adverse effect of a particular medication in causing an unpleasant hypersensitivity to alcohol, similar to the effect caused by disulfiram administration.

Examples:

- Antibiotics (nitroimidazoles), e.g. metronidazole
- First-generation sulfonylureas, e.g. tolbutamide and chlorpropamide
- Several cephalosporin drugs, including cefoperazone, cefamandole and cefotetan, that have a N-methylthio-tetrazole moiety
- Griseofulvin, an oral antifungal drug

- Procarbazine
- Temposil, or citrated calcium carbimide, has the same function as disulfiram, but is weaker and safer.
- Coprine, which metabolizes to 1-aminocyclopropanol, a chemical having the same metabolic effects as disulfiram. It occurs naturally in the otherwise edible common ink cap mushroom (*Coprinopsis atramentaria*), hence its colloquial name "tippler's bane". Similar reactions have been recorded with *Clitocybe clavipes* and *Suillellus luridus*, although the agent in those species is unknown.

History

This chemical and similar compounds were used in the vulcanization of rubber for tires, and it had been noted that workers in those industries often had adverse reactions to alcohol; the connection between the reaction and exposure to these chemicals, though, had not been deduced. However in 1948 researchers Erik Jacobsen, Jens Hald, and Keneth Ferguson at the Danish drug company Medicinalco uncovered the connection when they self-dosed with the chemical in the course of testing it as a possible anti-parasitic, and found themselves reacting violently to alcohol consumption.

Disulfiram is currently sold under the trade names Antabuse and Antabus, manufactured by Odyssey Pharmaceuticals.

Safety

Though the Occupational Safety and Health Administration (OSHA) in the US has not set a permissible exposure limit (PEL) for disulfiram in the workplace, the National Institute for Occupational Safety and Health has set a recommended exposure limit (REL) of 2 mg/m^3 and recommended that workers avoid concurrent exposure to ethylene dibromide.

Naltrexone

Naltrexone is a medication that stops the activity of opioids. It is primarily used in the management of alcohol dependence and opioid dependence.

The closely related medication, methylnaltrexone, is used to treat opioid-induced constipation but does not treat addiction as it does not cross the blood brain barrier. Nalmefene is similar to naltrexone and is used for the same purposes as naltrexone. Naltrexone should not be confused with naloxone, which is used in emergency cases of opioid overdose.

Naltrexone is marketed under the trade name Revia and Vivitrol. In the United States as of 2016, naltrexone tablets cost about US$0.91 per day. The extended-release injections cost about $1,248.50 per month ($41.62 per day). Naltrexone is also used in formulation with bupropion (bupropion/naltrexone) to treat obesity in the United States.

Medical Uses

Alcoholism

The main use of naltrexone is for the treatment of alcoholism. Naltrexone has been shown to decrease the amount and frequency of drinking. It does not appear to change the percentage of people drinking. Its overall benefit has been described as "modest".

Acamprosate may work better than naltrexone for eliminating drinking, while naltrexone may decrease the desire for alcohol to a greater extent.

The Sinclair method is a method of using opiate antagonists such as naltrexone to treat alcoholism. The patient takes the medication about an hour (and only then) before drinking to avoid side effects that arise from chronic use. The opioid blocks the positive reinforcement effects of alcohol and allows the person to stop or reduce drinking.

Opioid Use

Naltrexone helps patients overcome opioid addiction by blocking the effects of opioid drugs. It has little effect on opioid cravings. Naltrexone has in general been better studied for alcoholism than for opioids. It is more frequently used for alcoholism, despite its original approval by the FDA in 1984 for opioid addiction.

A 2011 review of studies suggested that naltrexone, when taken by mouth, was not superior to placebo or to no medication, nor was it superior to benzodiazepine or buprenorphine. Because of the poor quality of the reviewed studies, the authors found insufficient evidence to support naltrexone therapy when taken by mouth for an opioid use disorder. While some patients do well with the oral formulation, it must be taken daily, and a patient whose cravings become overwhelming can obtain opioid intoxication simply by skipping a dose. Due to this issue, the usefulness of oral naltrexone in opioid use disorders is limited by the low retention in treatment. Oral naltrexone remains an ideal treatment only for a small part of the opioid-addicted population, usually those with a stable social situation and motivation. With additional contingency management support, naltrexone is effective in a broader population.

Extended-release depot injections of naltrexone, administered once per month, have proven somewhat effective in treating opioid abuse, an approach that avoids the compliance issue that arises with oral formulations.

Adverse Effects

The most common side effects reported with naltrexone are gastrointestinal complaints such as diarrhea and abdominal cramping. These adverse effects are analogous to the symptoms of opioid withdrawal, as the mu receptor blockade will increase GI motility.

Naltrexone has been reported to cause liver damage (when given at doses higher than recommended). It carries an FDA boxed warning for this rare side effect. Due to these reports, some physicians may check liver function tests prior to starting naltrexone, and periodically thereafter. Concerns for liver toxicity initially arose from a study of non-addicted obese patients receiving 300 mg of naltrexone. Subsequent studies have suggested limited toxicity in other patient populations.

Naltrexone should not be started until several (typically 7-10) days of abstinence from opioids has been achieved. This is due to the risk of acute opioid withdrawal if naltrexone is taken, as naltrexone will displace most opioids from their receptors. The time of abstinence may be shorter than 7 days, depending on the half-life of the specific opioid taken. Some physicians use a naloxone challenge to determine whether an individual has any opioids remaining. The challenge involves giving a test dose of naloxone and monitoring for opioid withdrawal. If withdrawal occurs, naltrexone should not be started.

It is important that a person does not attempt to use opioids while using naltrexone. Although naltrexone blocks the opioid receptor, it is possible to override this blockade with high doses of opioids. This is quite dangerous, and may lead to opioid overdose, respiratory depression, and death. Similarly, a person will not show a normal response to opioid pain medications when taking naltrexone. In a supervised medical setting pain relief is possible, but may require higher than usual doses, and the individual should be closely monitored for respiratory depression. All individuals taking naltrexone are encouraged to keep a card or a note in their wallet in case of an injury or another medical emergency. This is to let medical personnel know that special procedures are required if opiate-based painkillers are to be used.

There has been some controversy regarding the use of opioid receptor antagonists such as naltrexone in the long-term management of opioid dependence, due to the effect of these agents in sensitizing opioid receptors. That is, after therapy, the opioid receptors continue to have increased sensitivity for a period during which the patient is at increased risk of opioid overdose. This effect reinforces the necessity of monitoring therapy, and provision of patient support measures by medical practitioners.

Contraindications

Naltrexone should not be used by persons with acute hepatitis or liver failure, or those with recent opioid use (typically 7–10 days).

Pharmacogenetics

A naltrexone treatment study by Anton et al., released by the National Institutes of Health in February 2008 and published in the *Archives of General Psychiatry*, has shown that alcoholics having a certain variant of the opioid receptor gene (G polymorphism of SNP Rs1799971 in the gene OPRM1), known as Asp40, demonstrated strong response to naltrexone and were far more likely to experience success at cutting back or discontinuing their alcohol intake altogether, while for those lacking the gene variant, naltrexone appeared to be no different from placebo. The G allele of OPRM1 is most common in individuals of Asian descent, with 60% to 70% of people of Chinese, Japanese, and Indian ancestry having at least one copy, as opposed to 30% of Europeans and few Africans.

Because of the characteristics of the patient group in the US, the first study was done on white patients and the next without regard for ethnicity. Anton et al. found that patients of African descent did not have much success with naltrexone in treatment for alcohol dependence because of lacking the relevant gene.

As white patients with the gene had a five times greater rate of success in reducing drinking when given naltrexone than did patients without the gene, when used in a protocol of Medical Management (MM).

"Because almost 25% of the treatment-seeking population carries the Asp40 allele, genetic testing of individuals before naltrexone treatment might be worth the cost and effort, especially if structured behavioral treatment were not being considered." This would enable treatment to be targeted by genetics to patients for whom it would be most effective. They noted, "Naltrexone is relatively easy to administer and free of serious adverse effects and, as we observed in the Asp40 carriers we studied, it appears to be highly effective."

Studies have found naltrexone to be more efficacious among certain white subjects, because of the genetic basis, than among black subjects, who generally do not carry the relevant gene variant. A 2009 study of naltrexone as an alcohol dependence treatment among African Americans failed to find any statistically significant differences between naltrexone and a placebo. Studies have suggested that carriers of the G allele may experience higher levels of craving and stronger "high" upon alcohol consumption, compared to carriers of the dominant allele, and naltrexone somewhat blunts these responses, leading to a reduction in alcohol use in some studies.

Mechanism of Action

Naltrexone and its active metabolite 6β-naltrexol are antagonists at the μ-opioid receptor (MOR), the κ-opioid receptor (KOR) to a lesser extent, and to a far lesser and possibly insignificant extent, at the δ-opioid receptor (DOR). The K_i affinity values of naltrexone at the MOR, KOR, and DOR have been reported as 0.0825 nM, 0.509 nM, and 8.02 nM, respectively, demonstrating a MOR/KOR binding ratio of 6.17 and a MOR/DOR binding ratio of 97.2.

The blockade of opioid receptors is the basis behind naltrexone's action in the management of opioid dependence—it reversibly blocks or attenuates the effects of opioids. Its mechanism of action in alcohol dependence is not fully understood, but as an opioid receptor antagonist is likely to be due to the modulation of the dopaminergic mesolimbic pathway (one of the primary centers for risk-reward analysis in the brain, and a tertiary "pleasure center") which is hypothesized to be a major center of the reward associated with addiction that all major drugs of abuse are believed to activate. Mechanism of action may be antagonism to endogenous opioids such as tetrahydropapaveroline, whose production is augmented in the presence of alcohol.

Structure and Pharmacokinetics

Naltrexone can be described as a substituted oxymorphone – here the tertiary amine methyl-substituent is replaced with methylcyclopropane. Naltrexone is the N-cyclopropylmethyl derivative of oxymorphone.

Naltrexone is metabolized mainly to 6β-naltrexol by the liver enzyme dihydrodiol dehydrogenase. Other metabolites include 2-hydroxy-3-methoxy-6β-naltrexol and 2-hydroxy-3-methoxy-naltrexone. These are then further metabolized by conjugation with glucuronide.

The plasma half-life of naltrexone and its metabolite 6β-naltrexol are about 4 hours and 13 hours, respectively.

Formulations

Vivitrol, a naltrexone formulation for depot injection, was approved by the FDA on April 13, 2006, for the treatment of alcohol dependence.

Additionally, naltrexone implants that are surgically implanted are available, although they are authorized for export only (i.e. not for use within Australia). By 2009, naltrexone implants showed encouraging results.

Controversies

Krupitsky et al 2011 Alkermes-funded Study

The FDA authorized use of injectable naltrexone (Vivitrol) for opioid addiction using a single study that was led by Evgeny Krupitsky MD at Bekhterev Research Psychoneurological Institute, St Petersburg State Pavlov Medical University, St Petersburg, Russia, a country where opioid agonists such as methadone and buprenorphine are not available. Krupitsky et al undertook a "double-blind, placebo-controlled, randomised", 24-week trial running "from July 3, 2008 through October 5, 2009" with "250 patients with opioid dependence disorder" at "13 clinical sites in Russia" on the use of injectable naltrexone (XR-NTX) for opioid dependence. The study was funded by the Boston-based biotech Alkermes firm which produces and markets naltrexone in the United

States. An 2011 article reported that this single trial of naltrexone was performed not by comparing it to the best available, evidence-based treatment (methadone or buprenorphine) but by comparing it with a placebo. In addition, the study failed to follow up on participants to document post-treatment overdose - a key measure for opioid substitution therapies. Furthermore, by 2011, Vivitrol cost about $1,100 a month, compared to $11 a month for generic naltrexone. A second 2011 article argued that these factors led to criticism of the study's design and ethics, and, by extension, of the FDA's approval of injectable naltrexone for opioid addiction based on this study.

Tom Price's Remarks 2017

In May 2017, United States Secretary of Health and Human Services Tom Price, praised [vivitrol] as the future of opioid addiction treatment after visiting the company's plant in Ohio. His remarks set off sharp criticism with almost 700 experts in the field of substance abuse submitting a letter to Price cautioning him about Vivitrol's "marketing tactics" and warning him that his comment "ignore widely accepted science". The experts pointed out that Vivitrol's competitors, buprenorphine and methadone, are "less expensive", "more widely used" and have been "rigorously studied".

Price had claimed that buprenorphine and methadone were "simply substitute"s for "illicit drugs" whereas according to the letter, "the substantial body of research evidence supporting these treatments is summarized in guidance from within your own agency, including the Substance Abuse and Mental Health Services Administration, the US Surgeon General, the National Institute on Drug Abuse, and the Centers for Disease Control and Prevention. To briefly summarize, buprenorphine and methadone have been demonstrated to be highly effective in managing the core symptoms of opioid use disorder, reducing the risk of relapse and fatal overdose, and encouraging long-term recovery."

According to a June 11, 2017 The New York Times article, Alkermes "has spent years coaxing, with a deft lobbying strategy that has targeted lawmakers and law enforcement officials. The company has spent millions of dollars on contributions to officials struggling to stem the epidemic of opioid abuse. It has also provided thousands of free doses to encourage the use of Vivitrol in jails and prisons, which have by default become major detox centers".

Research

Depersonalization/Derealization

Naltrexone is sometimes used in the treatment of dissociative symptoms such as depersonalization and derealization. Some studies suggest it might help. Other small, preliminary studies have also shown benefit. It is thought that blockade of the KOR by naltrexone and naloxone is responsible for their effectiveness in ameliorating depersonalization and derealization. Since these drugs are less efficacious in blocking the KOR relative to the MOR, higher dose than typically used seem to be necessary.

Low-dose Naltrexone

“Low-dose naltrexone” (LDN) describes the “off-label” use of naltrexone at low doses for diseases not related to chemical dependency or intoxication, such as multiple sclerosis. More research needs to be done before it can be recommended for clinical use.

Although there are scientific studies showing its efficacy in some conditions such as fibromyalgia, other, more dramatic claims for its use in conditions like cancer and HIV have less scientific support. This treatment has received significant attention on the Internet, especially through websites run by organizations promoting its use.

Tobacco Dependence

A study done by The Chicago Stop Smoking Research Project at the University of Chicago found that naltrexone did not help to improve a subject’s chance of attaining smoking cessation when compared to a placebo.

Self-injurious Behaviors

Some studies suggest that self-injurious behaviors present in persons with developmental disabilities (including autism) can sometimes be remedied with naltrexone. In these cases, it is believed that the self-injury is being done to release beta-endorphin, which binds to the same receptors as heroin and morphine. If the “rush” generated by self-injury is removed, the behavior may stop.

Behavioral Disorders

There are indications that naltrexone might be beneficial in the treatment of impulse control disorders such as kleptomania, compulsive gambling, or trichotillomania (compulsive hair pulling), but there is conflicting evidence of its effectiveness for gambling. A 2008 case study reported successful use of naltrexone in suppressing and treating an internet pornography addiction.

Countering Adverse Effects of Interferon Alpha

Naltrexone is effective in suppressing the cytokine-mediated adverse neuropsychiatric effects of interferon alpha therapy.

Drug Detoxification

Drug detoxification (informally, detox) is variously the intervention in a case of physical dependence to a drug; the process and experience of a withdrawal syndrome; and any of various treatments for acute drug overdose.

A detoxification program for physical dependence does not necessarily address the precedents of addiction, social factors, psychological addiction, or the often-complex behavioral issues that intermingle with addiction.

The United States Department of Health and Human Services acknowledges three steps in a drug detoxification process:

1. *Evaluation*: Upon beginning drug detoxification, a patient is first tested to see which specific substances are presently circulating in their bloodstream and the amount. Clinicians also evaluate the patient for potential co-occurring disorders, dual diagnosis, and mental/behavioral issues.

2. *Stabilization*: In this stage, the patient is guided through the process of detoxification. This may be done with or without the use of medications but for the most part the former is more common. Also part of stabilization is explaining to the patient what to expect during treatment and the recovery process. Where appropriate, people close to the addict are brought in at this time to become involved and show support.

3. *Guiding Patient into Treatment*: The last step of the detoxification process is to ready the patient for the actual recovery process. As drug detoxification only deals with the physical dependency and addiction to drugs, it does not address the psychological aspects of drug addiction. This stage entails obtaining agreement from the patient to complete the process by enrolling in a drug rehabilitation program.

Rapid Detoxification

The principle of rapid detoxification is to use heavy sedation alongside dosing with opioid antagonists. This approach is expensive, ineffective and extremely dangerous.

Origin of the Term

The concept of "detoxification" comes from the discredited autotoxin theory of George E. Pettey and others. David F. Musto says that "according to Pettey, opiates stimulated the production of toxins in the intestines, which had the physiological effect associated with withdrawal phenomena Therefore treatment would consist of purging the body of toxins and any lurking morphine that might remain to stimulate toxin production in the future."

Rapid Detox Controversy

Naltrexone therapy, which critics claim lacks long-term efficacy and can actually be detrimental to a patient's long-term recovery, has led to controversy. Additionally, there have been many questions raised about the ethics as well as safety of rapid detox following a number of deaths resulting from the procedure.

Drug Rehabilitation

Drug rehabilitation (often drug rehab or just rehab) is a term for the processes of medical or psychotherapeutic treatment, for dependency on psychoactive substances such as alcohol, prescription drugs, and street drugs such as cocaine, heroin or amphetamines. The general intent is to enable the patient to confront substance dependence, if present, and cease substance abuse in order to avoid the psychological, legal, financial, social, and physical consequences that can be caused, especially by extreme abuse. Treatment includes medication for depression or other disorders, counseling by experts and sharing of experience with other addicts. Some rehab centers include meditation and spiritual wisdom in the treatment process. A few centers also treat gambling with the same techniques as are used in drug rehabilitation.

Psychological Dependency

Psychological dependency is addressed in many drug rehabilitation programs by attempting to teach the patient new methods of interacting in a drug-free environment. In particular, patients are generally encouraged, or possibly even required, to not associate with friends who still use the addictive substance. Twelve-step programs encourage addicts not only to stop using alcohol or other drugs, but to examine and change habits related to their addictions. Many programs emphasize that recovery is a permanent process without culmination. For legal drugs such as alcohol, complete abstention—rather than attempts at moderation, which may lead to relapse—is also emphasized ("One is too many, and a thousand is never enough.") Whether moderation is achievable by those with a history of abuse remains a controversial point, but is generally considered unsustainable.

Types of Treatment

Various types of programs offer help in drug rehabilitation, including: residential treatment (in-patient), out-patient, local support groups, extended care centers, recovery or sober houses, addiction counselling, mental health, and medical care. Some rehab centers offer age- and gender-specific programs.

In a survey of treatment providers from three separate institutions (the National Association of Alcoholism and Drug Abuse Counselors, Rational Recovery Systems and the Society of Psychologists in Addictive Behaviors) measuring the treatment provider's responses on the Spiritual Belief Scale (a scale measuring belief in the four spiritual characteristics AA identified by Ernest Kurtz); the scores were found to explain 41% of the variance in the treatment provider's responses on the Addiction Belief Scale (a scale measuring adherence to the disease model or the free-will model addiction).

Scientific research since 1970 shows that effective treatment addresses the multiple needs of the patient rather than treating addiction alone. In addition, medically assisted drug detoxification or alcohol detoxification alone is ineffective as a treatment for addiction. The National Institute on Drug Abuse (NIDA) recommends detoxification followed by both medication (where applicable) and behavioral therapy, followed by relapse prevention. According to NIDA, effective treatment must address medical and mental health services as well as follow-up options, such as community or family based recovery support systems. Whatever the methodology, patient motivation is an important factor in treatment success.

For individuals addicted to prescription drugs, treatments tend to be similar to those who are addicted to drugs affecting the same brain systems. Medication like methadone and buprenorphine can be used to treat addiction to prescription opiates, and behavioral therapies can be used to treat addiction to prescription stimulants, benzodiazepines, and other drugs.

Types of behavioral therapy include:

- Cognitive-behavioral therapy, which seeks to help patients to recognize, avoid and cope with situations in which they are most likely to relapse.
- Multidimensional family therapy, which is designed to support recovery of the patient by improving family functioning.
- Motivational interviewing, which is designed to increase patient motivation to change behavior and enter treatment.
- Motivational incentives, which uses positive reinforcement to encourage abstinence from the addictive substance.

Medications

Certain opioid medications such as methadone and more recently buprenorphine (In America, "Subutex" and "Suboxone") are widely used to treat addiction and dependence on other opioids such as heroin, morphine or oxycodone. Methadone and buprenorphine are maintenance therapies intended to reduce cravings for opiates, thereby reducing illegal drug use, and the risks associated with it, such as disease, arrest, incarceration, and death, in line with the philosophy of harm reduction. Both drugs may be used as maintenance medications (taken for an indefinite period of time), or used as detoxification aids. All available studies collected in the 2005 Australian National Evaluation of Pharmacotherapies for Opioid Dependence suggest that maintenance treatment is preferable, with very high rates (79–100%) of relapse within three months of detoxification from LAAM, buprenorphine, and methadone.

Ibogaine is a hallucinogenic drug promoted by certain fringe groups to interrupt both physical dependence and psychological craving to a broad range or drugs including narcotics, stimulants, alcohol and nicotine. To date, there have never been any controlled studies showing it to be effective, and it is accepted as a treatment by no association of physicians, pharmacists, or addictionologists. There have been several deaths related to ibogaine use, which causes tachycardia and long QT syndrome. The drug is an illegal Schedule I controlled substance in the United States, and the foreign facilities in which it is administered tend to have little oversight, and range from motel rooms to one moderately-sized rehabilitation center. Some antidepressants also show usefulness in moderating drug use, particularly to nicotine, and it has become common for researchers to re-examine already approved drugs for new uses in drug rehabilitation.

According to the National Institute on Drug Abuse (NIDA), patients stabilized on adequate, sustained doses of methadone or buprenorphine can keep their jobs, avoid crime and violence, and reduce their exposure to HIV and Hepatitis C by stopping or reducing injection drug use and drug-related high risk sexual behavior. Naltrexone is a long-acting opioid antagonist with few side effects. It is usually prescribed in outpatient medical conditions. Naltrexone blocks the euphoric effects of alcohol and opiates. Naltrexone cuts relapse risk during the first 3 months by about 36%. However, it is far less effective in helping patients maintain abstinence or retaining them in the drug-treatment system (retention rates average 12% at 90 days for naltrexone, average 57% at 90 days for buprenorphine, average 61% at 90 days for methadone).

Acamprosate, disulfiram and topiramate (a novel anticonvulsant sulphonated sugar) are also used to treat alcohol addiction. Acamprosate has shown effectiveness for patients with severe dependence, helping them to maintain abstinence for several weeks or months. Disulfiram (also called Antabuse) produces a very unpleasant reaction when drinking alcohol that includes flushing, nausea and palpitations. It is more effective for patients with high motivation and some addicts use it only for high risk situations.

Nitrous oxide has been shown to be an effective treatment for a number of addictions.

Residential Treatment

In-patient residential treatment for alcohol abuse is expensive and common in the U.S. Most American programs follow a traditional 28-day program length. The length is based solely upon providers' experience in the 1940s that clients needed about one week to get over the physical changes, another week to understand the program, and another week or two to become stable. Seventy to 80 percent of American residential alcohol treatment programs provide 12-step therapy.

Experimental Treatment

The Nature of Things, a CBC Television program by David Suzuki, explored an experimental drug treatment by Dr. Gabor Maté who works with addicts in Vancouver which uses the substance Ayahuasca.

Criminal Justice

Drug rehabilitation is sometimes part of the criminal justice system. People convicted of minor drug offenses may be sentenced to rehabilitation instead of prison, and those convicted of driving while intoxicated are sometimes required to attend Alcoholics Anonymous meetings. There are a number of ways to address an alternative sentence in a drug possession or DUI case; increasingly, American courts are willing to explore outside-the-box methods for delivering this service. There have been lawsuits filed, and won, regarding the requirement of attending Alcoholics Anonymous and other twelve-step meetings as being inconsistent with the Establishment Clause of the First Amendment of the U. S. Constitution, mandating separation of church and state.

In some cases, individuals can be court ordered to drug rehabilitation by the state through legislation like the Marchman Act.

Counseling

Traditional addiction treatment is based primarily on counseling.

Counselors help individuals identifying behaviors and problems related to their addiction. It can be done on an individual basis, but it's more common to find it in a group setting and can include crisis counseling, weekly or daily counseling, and drop-in counseling supports. They are trained to develop recovery programs that help to reestablish healthy behaviors and provide coping strategies whenever a situation of risk happens. It's very common to see them work also with family members who are affected by the addictions of the individual, or in a community in order to prevent addiction and educate the public. Counselors should be able to recognize how addiction affects the whole person and those around him or her. Counseling is also related to "Intervention"; a process in which the addict's family requests help from a professional in order to get this person into drug treatment. This process begins with one of this professionals' first goals: breaking down denial of the person with the addiction. Denial implies lack of willingness from the patients or fear to confront the true nature of the addiction and to take any action to improve their lives, besides of continuing the destructive behavior. Once this has been achieved, professional coordinates with the addict's family to support them on getting this family member to alcohol drug rehabilitation immediately, with concern and care for this person. Otherwise, this person will be asked to leave and expect no support of any kind until going into drug rehabilitation or alcoholism treatment. An intervention can also be conducted in the workplace environment with colleagues instead of family.

One approach with limited applicability is the Sober Coach. In this approach, the client is serviced by provider(s) in his or her home and workplace — for any efficacy, around-the-clock — who functions much like a nanny to guide or control the patient's behavior.

Twelve-step Programs

The disease model of addiction has long contended the maladaptive patterns of alcohol and substance use displayed by addicted individuals are the result of a lifelong disease that is biological in origin and exacerbated by environmental contingencies. This conceptualization renders the individual essentially powerless over his or her problematic behaviors and unable to remain sober by himself or herself, much as individuals with a terminal illness are unable to fight the disease by themselves without medication. Behavioral treatment, therefore, necessarily requires individuals to admit their addiction, renounce their former lifestyle, and seek a supportive social network who can help them remain sober. Such approaches are the quintessential features of Twelve-step programs, originally published in the book Alcoholics Anonymous in 1939. These approaches have met considerable amounts of criticism, coming from opponents who disapprove of the spiritual-religious orientation on both psychological and legal grounds. Nonetheless, despite this criticism, outcome studies have revealed that affiliation with twelve-step programs predicts abstinence success at 1-year follow-up for alcoholism. Different results have been reached for other drugs, with the twelve steps being less beneficial for addicts to illicit substances, and least beneficial to those addicted to the physiologically and psychologically addicting opioids, for which maintenance therapies are the gold standard of care.

Client-centered Approaches

In his influential book, *Client-Centered Therapy*, in which he presented the client-centered approach to therapeutic change, psychologist Carl Rogers proposed there are three necessary and sufficient conditions for personal change: unconditional positive regard, accurate empathy, and genuineness. Rogers believed the presence of these three items in the therapeutic relationship could help an individual overcome any troublesome issue, including alcohol abuse. To this end, a 1957 study compared the relative effectiveness of three different psychotherapies in treating alcoholics who had been committed to a state hospital for sixty days: a therapy based on two-factor learning theory, client-centered therapy, and psychoanalytic therapy. Though the authors expected the two-factor theory to be the most effective, it actually proved to be deleterious in outcome. Surprisingly, client-centered therapy proved most effective. It has been argued, however, these findings may be attributable to the profound difference in therapist outlook between the two-factor and client-centered approaches, rather than to client-centered techniques per se. The authors note two-factor theory involves stark disapproval of the clients' "irrational behavior"; this notably negative outlook could explain the results.

A variation of Rogers' approach has been developed in which clients are directly responsible for determining the goals and objectives of the treatment. Known as Client-Directed Outcome-Informed therapy (CDOI), this approach has been utilized by several drug treatment programs, such as Arizona's Department of Health Services.

Psychoanalysis

Psychoanalysis, a psychotherapeutic approach to behavior change developed by Sigmund Freud and modified by his followers, has also offered an explanation of substance abuse. This orientation suggests the main cause of the addiction syndrome is the unconscious need to entertain and to enact various kinds of homosexual and perverse fantasies, and at the same time to avoid taking responsibility for this. It is hypothesised specific drugs facilitate specific fantasies and using drugs is considered to be a displacement from, and a concomitant of, the compulsion to masturbate while entertaining homosexual and perverse fantasies. The addiction syndrome is also hypothesised to be associated with life trajectories that have occurred within the context of traumatogenic processes, the phases of which include social, cultural and political factors, encapsulation, traumatophilia, and masturbation as a form of self-soothing. Such an approach lies in stark contrast to the approaches of social cognitive theory to addiction—and indeed, to behavior in general—which holds human beings regulate and control their own environmental and cognitive environments, and are not merely driven by internal, driving impulses. Additionally, homosexual content is not implicated as a necessary feature in addiction.

Relapse Prevention

An influential cognitive-behavioral approach to addiction recovery and therapy has been Alan Marlatt's (1985) Relapse Prevention approach. Marlatt describes four psychosocial processes relevant to the addiction and relapse processes: self-efficacy, outcome expectancies, attributions of causality, and decision-making processes. Self-efficacy refers to one's ability to deal competently and effectively with high-risk, relapse-provoking situations. Outcome expectancies refer to an individual's expectations about the psychoactive effects of an addictive substance. Attributions of causality refer to an individual's pattern of beliefs that relapse to drug use is a result of internal, or rather external, transient causes (e.g., allowing oneself to make exceptions when faced with what are judged to be unusual circumstances). Finally, decision-making processes are implicated in the relapse process as well. Substance use is the result of multiple decisions whose collective effects result in consumption of the intoxicant. Furthermore, Marlatt stresses some decisions—referred to as apparently irrelevant decisions—may seem inconsequential to relapse, but may actually have downstream implications that place the user in a high-risk situation.

For example: As a result of heavy traffic, a recovering alcoholic may decide one afternoon to exit the highway and travel on side roads. This will result in the creation of a high-risk situation when he realizes he is inadvertently driving by his old favorite bar. If this individual is able to employ successful coping strategies, such as distracting himself from his cravings by turning on his favorite music, then he will avoid the relapse risk (PATH 1) and heighten his efficacy for future abstinence. If, however, he lacks coping mechanisms—for instance, he may begin ruminating on his cravings (PATH

2)—then his efficacy for abstinence will decrease, his expectations of positive outcomes will increase, and he may experience a lapse—an isolated return to substance intoxication. So doing results in what Marlatt refers to as the Abstinence Violation Effect, characterized by guilt for having gotten intoxicated and low efficacy for future abstinence in similar tempting situations. This is a dangerous pathway, Marlatt proposes, to full-blown relapse.

Cognitive Therapy

An additional cognitively-based model of substance abuse recovery has been offered by Aaron Beck, the father of cognitive therapy and championed in his 1993 book, Cognitive Therapy of Substance Abuse. This therapy rests upon the assumption addicted individuals possess core beliefs, often not accessible to immediate consciousness (unless the patient is also depressed). These core beliefs, such as "I am undesirable," activate a system of addictive beliefs that result in imagined anticipatory benefits of substance use and, consequentially, craving. Once craving has been activated, permissive beliefs ("I can handle getting high just this one more time") are facilitated. Once a permissive set of beliefs have been activated, then the individual will activate drug-seeking and drug-ingesting behaviors. The cognitive therapist's job is to uncover this underlying system of beliefs, analyze it with the patient, and thereby demonstrate its dysfunctionality. As with any cognitive-behavioral therapy, homework assignments and behavioral exercises serve to solidify what is learned and discussed during treatment.

Emotion Regulation and Mindfulness

A growing literature is demonstrating the importance of emotion regulation in the treatment of substance abuse. Considering that nicotine and other psychoactive substances such as cocaine activate similar psychopharmacological pathways, an emotion regulation approach may be applicable to a wide array of substance abuse. Proposed models of affect-driven tobacco use have focused on negative reinforcement as the primary driving force for addiction; according to such theories, tobacco is used because it helps one escape from the undesirable effects of nicotine withdrawal or other negative moods. Acceptance and commitment therapy (ACT), is showing evidence that it is effective in treating substance abuse, including the treatment of poly-substance abuse and cigarette smoking. Mindfulness programs that encourage patients to be aware of their own experiences in the present moment and of emotions that arise from thoughts, appear to prevent impulsive/compulsive responses. Research also indicates that mindfulness programs can reduce the consumption of substances such as alcohol, cocaine, amphetamines, marijuana, cigarettes and opiates.

Behavioral Models

Behavioral models make use of principles of functional analysis of drinking behavior. Behavior models exists for both working with the substance abuser (Community Reinforcement Approach) and their family (Community Reinforcement Approach and Family Training). Both these models have had considerable research success for both efficacy and effectiveness. This model lays much emphasis on the use of problem solving techniques as a means of helping the addict to overcome his addiction.

Recovery Coaching

Recovery coaching is a form of strengths-based support for persons with addictions or in recovery from alcohol, other drugs, codependency, or other addictive behaviors. Recovery coaches work with persons with active addictions as well as persons already in recovery. Recovery coaches are helpful for making decisions about what to do with one's life and the part addiction or recovery plays in it. Recovery coaches help clients find ways to stop addiction (abstinence), or reduce harm associated with addictive behaviors. Recovery coaches can help a client find resources for harm reduction, detox, treatment, family support and education, local or online support groups; or help a client create a change plan to recover on their own.

Recovery coaches do not offer primary treatment for addiction, do not diagnose, and are not associated with any particular method or means of recovery. Recovery coaches support any positive change, helping persons coming home from treatment to avoid relapse, build community support for recovery, or work on life goals not related to addiction such as relationships, work, education etc. Recovery coaching is action oriented with an emphasis on improving present life and reaching goals for the future.

Recovery coaching is unlike most therapy because coaches do not address the past, do not work to heal trauma, and there is little emphasis on feelings. Recovery coaches are unlike licensed addiction counselors in that coaches are non-clinical and do not diagnose or treat addiction or any mental health issues.

Relationship to Life Coaching

Similar to life and business coaching, recovery coaching use a partnership model wherein the client is considered to be the expert on his or her life, the one who decides what is worth doing, and the coach provides expertise in supporting successful change. Recovery coaching focuses on achieving any goals important to the client—not just recovery-related goals. The coach asks questions and offers reflections to help the client reach clarity and decide what steps to take. Recovery coaching emphasizes honoring values and making principle-based decisions, creating a clear plan of action, and using current strengths to reach future goals. The coach provides accountability to help the client stay on track.

Other Similar Terms

The moniker "recovery coach" is used for a variety specific addiction support roles. The main distinction is between the professional or highly compensated Recovery Coach and the volunteer or agency employed Peer Recovery Support Specialist. Recovery support roles include the following:

Sober escort-a paid sober travel companion or travel escort that accompanies a client to an event, to treatment, to court and insures sobriety.Transportation can be a significant challenge to a newly abstinent person. Whether the client is interested in maintaining an ongoing recovery or just needs to stay abstinent for a period of time, getting from point A to point B can be difficult. Commonly called Travel Escorts or Sober Escorts, this version of a recovery coach may be required to transport a person in recovery across town, across the state, or across the county.

Many clients are introduced to a Travel or Sober Escort after an intervention, when immediate transportation to a treatment center is required. In the event a client is in a treatment center and a death in the family occurs, or they must appear in court, a Travel or Sober Escort will safely transport the client to and from the specific event safely. When a client is ready to leave a treatment center and return home, a Travel or Sober Escort will safely transport the client home.

Sober companion or sober coach. A sober companion works "full-time" with the client: full work days, nights, weekends or extended periods where the coach is by the client's side 24 hours a day. Some recovery coach roles have evolved from a travel or sober escort to a Long Term Recovery Coach or Sober Companion. A Long Term Recovery Coach or Sober Companion works "full-time" with the client: full work days, nights, weekends or extended periods where the coach is by the client's side 24 hours a day. This long term option can begin with treatment discharge, the client's first day or weekend home and may develop into a coaching relationship that continues for several weeks, months or longer.

Returning home from treatment, the client trades a secure, drug-free environment for a situation where they know there are problems. A Long Term Recovery Coach or Sober Companion will provide the symbolic and functional safety of the treatment center. A Long Term Recovery Coach or Sober Companion will introduce the client to 12 step meetings; guide them past former triggers (e.g. liquor stores or strip clubs) and support the client in developing their recovery plan. A Long Term Recovery Coach or Sober Companion will help the client to make lifestyle changes in order to experience a better quality of life in the first crucial days after discharge from a treatment center. Sometimes a recovery coach is necessary to keep a client sober in order to regain custody of their child.

Recovery support specialist (RSS) – a recovery support specialist(RSS) or a peer recovery support specialist (PRSS) is a non-clinical person who meets with clients in a recovery community organization, or goes off sight to visit a client. The Recovery Support Specialist may volunteer for these coaching services or be employed by a recovery community organization at minimum wage or slightly higher. The recovery support specialist ensures there is a contract for engagement, called a personal recovery plan. A key component of the Recovery Management model that all RSS follow, is this personal recovery plan. Peer Recovery support specialists (PRSS) are sometimes called "recovery coaches". William L. White long standing researcher and original author of the recovery management model, uses the term "recovery support specialist" and this is referenced in the paper entitled: Recovery Oriented System of Care (ROSC) Substance Use Disorder (SUD) Glossary of Terms, compiled by the Bureau of Substance Abuse and Addiction Services (BSAAS). Other terms used to describe peer recovery support specialist is a peer mentor.

Family Recovery Coach – The family plays such an important role for a person in recovery, yet is so often neglected by traditional models of recovery. Specially trained Family Recovery Coaches strive to create a calm, objective, non-judgmental environment for the family of a recovering addict. These coaches are knowledgeable in specific models that aid the family coping with the changes that they have gone through living with an active addict or living with a recovering addict. Regardless of an addict's choices, working with a Family Recovery Coach helps a spouse; partner; or loved ones avoid the mental obsession that plagues so many families affected by addiction and learn to lead sane and productive lives (Buncher, 2012).

Telephone or Virtual Recovery Coach – A Telephone or Virtual Recovery Coaching relationship may be established to continue beyond the face to face meeting of a client and a recovery coach, sober escort or a sober companion coach. The prior face to face coaching relationship was built on trust and re-established honesty for the client, so the Telephone or Virtual Recovery Coach relationship can continue in the same light, with daily or weekly telephone or web based conversations (Bronfman, Fisher, Gilbert & Valentine 2006).

Today, many treatment centers are embracing virtual recovery coaching and linking Telephone or Virtual Recovery Coaches to clients prior to leaving treatment as a way to continue the connection to the treatment center, as well as meeting guidelines of an 'aftercare' program. On line virtual coaching programs has also sprung up recently, either fee based or for free, that will help anyone apply the methods of recovery (e.g. developing a recovery plan and building recovery capital) whether the person has departed from a 30-day stay at a treatment center or relapsed many months after treatment.

Legal Support Specialist – Recovery Coach – Recently, lawyers dealing with criminal drug cases or drug courts have been requesting a type of recovery coaching to ensure a client, (perhaps under house arrest, enrolled in a drug court outpatient program or pending trial) stays sober as per the law's mandate. Recovery Coaches with the required certification and legal knowledge are contracted for this purpose. Coaches licensed as a Licensed Clinical Social Worker or Certified Alcohol and Drug Counselor with training in assessments can perform these tasks. The courts request them to perform a client assessment. The coach will then draft a letter to the court and offer suggested placement in a residential alcohol/drug treatment center, an outpatient treatment program and/ or a sober living facility. A Legal Support Specialist – Recovery Coach can also appear in court with the client and provide transportation to or from courthouse, Bob Timmins acted as a legal support specialist/recovery coach for many clients in his capacity in the California Drug Court system.

Brief History

In 1984, the rock group Aerosmith was attempting a comeback; but it was not working, just as their newest album Back in the Saddle was not climbing the charts. There were a lot of things that were not working for Aerosmith, Joe Perry and Steven Tyler, front men for the group, are referred to as the "Toxic Twins" for their heroin habits and other behaviors on and off the stage. In fact, the entire band was heavily drinking or taking drugs.

That summer, while touring for the new album, co-manager, David Krebs, hired a psychiatrist to tour with the band. After a month, the doctor claimed the band was "unfixable". Krebs left the band. Aerosmith denied drugs were dragging down the tour and the album sales. (Aerosmith and Davis, 1997). The band pointed their fingers outward, blaming everyone else for their problems. The band changed record labels from CBS Records to Arista Records, and hired Tim Collins to manage the band.

Tim Collins, told the group that in order to survive they had to get sober, claiming that if they stopped using alcohol and drugs, he could take them "platinum" again. Band members Joey Kramer and Tom Hamilton both became sober and by the fall of 1986. Steven Tyler went to an in-treatment drug rehabilitation center, followed by Joe Perry. By the end of 1986, the final band member Brad Whitford had accepted sobriety. Even so, Aerosmith's sobriety commitment to Tim Collins was only partially completed. Collins still had to get these heavy metal rockers on the road, with roadies, groupies, opening acts and exposure to more drugs and alcohol, in order to promote their newest album, Permanent Vacation. Tim was able to help the group, maintain sobriety throughout the tour by contracting a recovery coach, Bob Timmins to stay with the band through the tour. A new era in recovery coaching had begun.

Recovery Coaching became more developed and professional in 2003 as a professional life-coaching niche. Alida Schuyler, a coach credentialed by the International Coach Federation (ICF) and a woman in recovery from addiction wrote the first recovery coach certification training program specifically aimed at training students to coach persons with addictions. She also created the first special interest group for recovery coaches, and she co-founded the nonprofit Recovery Coaches International with Andrew Susskind.

William L. White used the term "recovery coach" in his 2006 paper *Sponsor, Recovery Coach, Addiction Counselor* but later changed adopted the term "Peer Recovery

Support Specialist" to emphasize a community-based peer model of addiction support. Many recovery coaches use different recovery approaches adapted from the Minnesota Model. White's Recovery Management model adapted from the Minnesota Model includes recovery coaching (peer recovery support specialist) and was developed by William White in 2006. Alida Schuyler developed a professional model of life coaching for addiction recovery by blending the Minnesota Model and Harm Reduction model with the core competencies of the International Coach Federation (ICF).

Through the research completed by William White, David Loveland, Ernest Kurtz, Mark Saunders and the efforts funded through Faces and Voices of Recovery, the Fayette Companies, Great Lakes Addiction Technology Transfer Center, the Chestnut Health Systems and many other universities, research on recovery coaching is multiplying at a very rapid rate. Two research papers were published in 2009 and 2011 by Melissa Killeen and is housed at the University of Pennsylvania (PA) Library. Through this research the theory has been developed that recovery coaching reduces relapse by providing the recovering individual ongoing support developing healthy problem-solving skills and self efficacy (reaching worthwhile goals) as well as connecting with the local recovery community for additional support. In other words, recovery coaching helps the client develop the cognitive skills necessary for considering options and consequences, making clear choices, planning and taking actions toward healthier life and recovery goals. Recovery coaching is currently offered by such notable 12-step treatment centers as Hazelden through their MORE program.

In 2013, the first self-help book to offer readers Recovery Coaching techniques to help them rebuild their lives after addiction was published. *The Happy Addict: How to be Happy in Recovery from Alcoholism or Drug Addiction* (ISBN 978-0957321717), authored by Recovery Coach Beth Burgess, was released by Eightball Publishing in July 2013.

Addiction Recovery Support Groups

Recovery coaches encourage (but most do not require) participation in groups such as Alcoholics Anonymous (AA), Narcotics Anonymous (NA), Al-Anon or non 12-step groups such as LifeRing Secular Recovery, SMART Recovery, Moderation Management (MM), and Women for Sobriety. Recovery coaches do work with individuals who dislike groups to help them find their own path to recovery.

Niches within Recovery Coaching

Recovery coaches may work with any type of addict, an alcoholic, a drug addict, a gambler, a sex addict, a kleptomaniac, an over spender, absolutely any form of addiction. There are also niches within recovery coaching such as the coach that works exclusively with families of recovering individuals, or the financial coach that works on rebuilding an over spender's credit rating. There is a strong emphasis with peer recovery support specialists working with individuals that have left the prison system and are attempting to rebuild their lives, and there are recovery coaches who specialize in emotional and financial recovery from divorce.

There are also those few that specialize in essentially merging the characteristics of recovery coaching within a life coaching framework as described by Alexandra Birenbaum, MA, CAP, Life Coach & CSAT Candidate. The concept takes into account the often overlooked reality that those in early recovery tend to have unique difficulties in applying the realities of day-to-day living within their new sober lifestyle. Such unique coaching styles are able to span far beyond the recovery component and properly introduce outside influencers such as; family relations, work/employment, schooling, relationships, etc.

For those requiring a higher level of care, such as medical detoxification for heroin or opiate withdrawal for instance, or 24/7 sober companion and oversight services, there exists recovery coaching firms which specialize in providing what could often be described as an alternative to inpatient our outpatient treatment. Companies like The Addictions Coach and others which have nationwide credentials are able to essentially bring the addiction treatment component to the client, no matter where he or she may be located.

What Recovery Coaches Do

Recovery coaches support the client in achieving and maintaining a solid foundation in recovery, and building upon recovery to achieve other life goals that make recovery worthwhile. David Loveland and Michael Boyle wrote a lengthy manual on Recovery Coaching and how to guide an individual through creating their recovery plan William White, preeminent scholar on addictions, worked closely with the Philadelphia community based recovery center, PRO-ACT, to prepare a document outlining the "Ethical Guidelines for the Delivery of Peer-Based Recovery Support Services", (Faces and Voices of Recovery.org, 2007). These documents provide a discussion of what a recovery coach does. Also included in these guidelines are the definition of coaching roles as they relate to others in the realm of personal conduct and conduct in service relationships with the community service provider or treatment team. This document presents a simple statement of core competencies (Faces and Voices of Recovery.org, 2007).

Dual Diagnosis

Dual diagnosis (also called co-occurring disorders, COD) is the condition of suffering from a mental illness and a comorbid substance abuse problem. There is considerable debate surrounding the appropriateness of using a single category for a heterogeneous group of individuals with complex needs and a varied range of problems. The concept can be used broadly, for example depression and alcoholism, or it can be restricted to specify severe mental illness (e.g. psychosis, schizophrenia) and substance misuse disorder (e.g. cannabis abuse), or a person who has a milder mental illness and a drug dependency, such as panic disorder or generalized anxiety disorder and is dependent on opioids. Diagnosing a primary psychiatric illness in substance abusers is challenging as drug abuse itself often induces psychiatric symptoms, thus making it necessary to differentiate between substance induced and pre-existing mental illness.

Those with co-occurring disorders face complex challenges. They have increased rates of relapse, hospitalization, homelessness, and HIV and hepatitis C infection compared to those with either mental or substance use disorders alone. The cause of co-occurring disorders is unknown, although there are several theories.

Differentiating Pre-existing and Substance Induced

Drug abuse, including alcohol and prescription drugs, can induce symptomatology which resembles mental illness, which can make it difficult to differentiate between substance induced psychiatric syndromes and pre-existing mental health problems. More often than not psychiatric disorders among drug or alcohol abusers disappear with prolonged abstinence. Substance induced psychiatric symptoms can occur both in the intoxicated state and also during the withdrawal state. In some cases these substance induced psychiatric disorders can persist long after detoxification, such as prolonged psychosis or depression after amphetamine or cocaine abuse. Abuse of hallucinogens can trigger delusional and other psychotic phenomena long after cessation of use and cannabis may trigger panic attacks during intoxication and with use it may cause a state similar to dysthymia. Severe anxiety and depression are commonly induced by sustained alcohol abuse which in most cases abates with prolonged abstinence. Even moderate sustained use of alcohol may increase anxiety and depression levels in some individuals. In most cases these drug induced psychiatric disorders fade away with prolonged abstinence. A protracted withdrawal syndrome can also occur with psychiatric and other symptoms persisting for months after cessation of use. Benzodiazepines are the most notable drug for inducing prolonged withdrawal effects with symptoms sometimes persisting for years after cessation of use.

Prevalence

The 2011 USA National Survey on Drug Use and Health found that 17.5% of adults with a mental illness had a co-occurring substance use disorder; this works out to 7.98 million people. Estimates of co-occurring disorders in Canada are even higher, with an estimated 40-60% of adults with a severe and persistent mental illness experiencing a substance use disorder in their lifetime.

A study by Kessler et al. in the United States attempting to assess the prevalence of dual diagnosis found that 47% of clients with schizophrenia had a substance misuse disorder at some time in their life, and the chances of developing a substance misuse disorder was significantly higher among patients suffering from a psychotic illness than in those without a psychotic illness.

Another study looked at the extent of substance misuse in a group of 187 chronically mentally ill patients living in the community. According to the clinician's ratings, around a third of the sample used alcohol, street drugs, or both during the six months before evaluation.

Further UK studies have shown slightly more moderate rates of substance misuse among mentally ill individuals. One study found that individuals suffering from schizophrenia showed just a 7% prevalence of problematic drug use in the year prior to being interviewed and 21% reported problematic use some time before that.

Wright and colleagues identified individuals with psychotic illnesses who had been in contact with services in the London borough of Croydon over the previous 6 months. Cases of alcohol or substance misuse and dependence were identified through standardized interviews with clients and keyworkers. Results showed that prevalence rates of dual diagnosis were 33% for the use of any substance, 20% for alcohol misuse only and 5% for drug misuse only. A lifetime history of any illicit drug use was observed in 35% of the sample.

Diagnosis

Substance use disorders can be confused with other psychiatric disorders. There are diagnoses for substance-induced mood disorders and substance-induced anxiety disorders and thus such overlap can be complicated. For this reason, the DSM-IV advises that diagnoses of primary psychiatric disorders not be made in the absence of sobriety (of duration sufficient to allow for any substance-induced post-acute-withdrawal symptoms to dissipate) up to 1 year.

Treatment

Only a small proportion of those with co-occurring disorders actually receive treatment for both disorders. In 2011, it was estimated that only 12.4% of American adults with co-occurring disorders were receiving both mental health and addictions treatment. Clients with co-occurring disorders face challenges accessing treatment, as they may be excluded from mental health services if they admit to a substance abuse problem, and vice versa.

There are multiple approaches to treating concurrent disorders. Partial treatment involves treating only the disorder that is considered primary. Sequential treatment involves treating the primary disorder first, and then treating the secondary disorder after the primary disorder has been stabilized. Parallel treatment involves the client receiving mental health services from one provider, and addictions services from another.

Integrated treatment involves a seamless blending of interventions into a single coherent treatment package developed with a consistent philosophy and approach among care providers. With this approach, both disorders are considered primary. Integrated treatment can improve accessibility, service individualization, engagement in treatment, treatment compliance, mental health symptoms, and overall outcomes. The Substance Abuse and Mental Health Services Administration in the United States describes integrated treatment as being in the best interests or clients, programs, funders, and systems. Green suggested that treatment should be integrated, and a collaborative process between the treatment team and the patient. Furthermore, recovery should to be viewed as a marathon rather than a sprint, and methods and outcome goals should be explicit.

Although many patients may reject medications as antithetical to substance-abuse recovery and side effects, they can be useful to reduce paranoia, anxiety, and craving. Medications that have proven effective include opioid replacement therapies, such as lifelong maintenance on methadone or buprenorphine, to minimize risk of relapse, fatality, and legal trouble amongst opioid addicts, as well as helping with cravings, baclofen for alcoholics, opioid addicts, cocaine addicts, and amphetamine addicts, to help eliminate drug cravings, and clozapine, the first atypical antipsychotic, which appears to reduce illicit drug use amongst stimulant addicts. Clozapine can cause respiratory arrest when combined with alcohol, benzodiazepines, or opioids, so it is not recommended to use in these groups.

Theories of Dual Diagnosis

There are a number of theories that explain the relationship between mental illness and substance abuse.

Causality

The causality theory suggests that certain types of substance abuse may causally lead to mental illness.

There is strong evidence that using cannabis can produce temporary and usually mild psychotic and affective experiences. When it comes to persisting effects, there is a clear increase in incidence of psychotic outcomes in people who had used cannabis, even when they had used it only once. More frequent use of cannabis strongly augmented the risk for psychosis. The evidence for affective outcomes is less strong. However, this connection between cannabis and psychosis does not prove that cannabis *causes* psychotic disorders. The causality theory for cannabis has been challenged as despite explosive increases in cannabis consumption over the past 40 years in western society, the rate of schizophrenia (and psychosis in general) has remained relatively stable.

Attention-deficit Hyperactivity Disorder

One in four people who have a substance use disorder also have attention-deficit hyperactivity disorder, which makes the treatment of both conditions more difficult. ADHD is associated with an increased craving for drugs. Having ADHD makes it more likely that an individual will initiate substance misuse at a younger age than their peers. They are also more likely to have a poorer outcome, such as longer time to remission, and increased psychiatric complications from substance misuse. While generally stimulant medications do not seem to worsen substance misuse, they are known to be abused in some cases. Psychosocial therapy and/or nonstimulant medications and extended release stimulants are ADHD treatment options that reduce these risks.

Autism Spectrum Disorder

Unlike ADHD, which significantly increases the risk of substance use disorder, autism spectrum disorder has the opposite effect of significantly reducing the risk of substance abuse. This is because introversion, inhibition and lack of sensation seeking personality traits, which are typical of autism spectrum disorder, protect against substance abuse and thus substance abuse levels are low in individuals who are on the autism spectrum. However, certain forms of substance abuse, especially alcohol abuse, can cause or worsen certain neuropsychological symptoms which are common to autism spectrum disorder, such as impaired social skills due to the neurotoxic effects of alcohol on the brain, especially the prefrontal cortex area of the brain. The social skills that are impaired by alcohol abuse include impairments in perceiving facial emotions, prosody perception problems and theory of mind deficits; the ability to understand humour is also impaired in alcohol abusers.

Past Exposure to Psychiatric Medications Theory

The past exposure theory suggests that exposure to psychiatric medication alters neural synapses, introducing an imbalance that was not previously present. Discontinuation of the drug is expected to result in symptoms of psychiatric illness which resolve once the drug is restarted. This theory suggests that while it may appear that the medication is working, it is only treating a disorder caused by the medication itself. New exposure to psychiatric medication may lead to heightened sensitivity to the effects of drugs and alcohol, which has a deteriorating effect on the patient.

Self-medication Theory

The self-medication theory suggests that people with severe mental illnesses misuse substances in order to relieve a specific set of symptoms and counter the negative side-effects of antipsychotic medication.

Khantizan proposes that substances are not randomly chosen, but are specifically selected for their effects. For example, using stimulants such as nicotine or amphetamines can be used to combat the sedation that can be caused by higher doses of certain types of (usually typical) antipsychotic medication. Conversely, some people taking medications with a stimulant effect such as the SNRI antidepressants Effexor (venlafaxine) or

Wellbutrin (bupropion) may seek out benzodiazepines or opioid narcotics to counter the anxiety and insomnia that such medications sometimes evoke.

Some studies show that nicotine administration can be effective for reducing motor side-effects of antipsychotics, with both bradykinesia (stiff muscles) and dyskinesia(involuntary movement) being prevented.

Alleviation of Dysphoria Theory

The alleviation of dysphoria theory suggests that people with severe mental illness commonly have a negative self-image, which makes them vulnerable to using psychoactive substances to alleviate these feelings. Despite the existence of a wide range of dysphoric feelings (anxiety, depression, boredom, and loneliness), the literature on self-reported reasons for use seems to lend support for the experience of these feelings being the primary motivator for drug and alcohol misuse.

Multiple Risk Factor Theory

Another theory is that there may be shared risk factors that can lead to both substance abuse and mental illness. Mueser hypothesizes that these may include factors such as social isolation, poverty, lack of structured daily activity, lack of adult role responsibility, living in areas with high drug availability, and association with people who already misuse drugs.

Other evidence suggests that traumatic life events, such as sexual abuse, are associated with the development of psychiatric problems and substance abuse.

The Supersensitivity Theory

The supersensitivity theory proposes that certain individuals who have severe mental illness also have biological and psychological vulnerabilities, caused by genetic and early environmental life events. These interact with stressful life events and can result in either a psychiatric disorder or trigger a relapse into an existing illness. The theory states that although anti-psychotic medication can reduce the vulnerability, substance abuse may increase it, causing the individual to be more likely to experience negative consequences from using relatively small amounts of substances. These individuals, therefore, are “supersensitive” to the effects of certain substances, and individuals with psychotic illness such as schizophrenia may be less capable of sustaining moderate substance use over time without experiencing negative symptoms.

Although there are limitations in the research studies conducted in this area, namely that most have focused primarily on schizophrenia, this theory provides an explanation of why relatively low levels of substance misuse often result in negative consequences for individuals with severe mental illness.

History

The traditional method for treating patients suffering from dual diagnosis was a parallel treatment program. In this format, patients received mental health services from one clinician while addressing their substance abuse with a separate clinician. However, researchers found that parallel treatments were ineffective, suggesting a need to integrate the services addressing mental health with those addressing substance abuse.

During the mid-1980s, a number of initiatives began to combine mental health and substance abuse services in an attempt to meet this need. These programs worked to shift the method of treatment for substance abuse from a confrontational approach to a supportive one. They also introduced new methods to motivate clients and worked with them to develop long-term goals for their care. Although the studies conducted by these initiatives did not have control groups, their results were promising and became the basis for more rigorous efforts to study and develop models of integrated treatment.

Nicotine Replacement Therapy

Nicotine replacement therapy (NRT) is a medically-approved way to take nicotine by means other than tobacco. It is used to help with quitting smoking or stopping chewing tobacco. It increases the chance of quitting smoking by about 50% to 70%. Often it is used along with other behavioral techniques. NRT has also been used to treat ulcerative colitis. Types of NRT include the adhesive patch, chewing gum, lozenges, nose spray, and inhaler. The use of more than one type of NRT at a time may increase effectiveness.

Common side effects depend on the formulation of nicotine. Common side effects with the gum include nausea, hiccups, and irritation of the mouth. Common side effects with the patch include skin irritation and a dry mouth while the inhaler commonly results in a cough, runny nose, or headaches. Serious risks include nicotine poisoning and continued addiction. They do not appear to increase the risk of heart attacks. There are possible harms to the baby if used during pregnancy. Nicotine replacement therapy works by reducing cravings due to nicotine addiction.

They were first approved for use in the United States in 1984. Nicotine replacement products are on the World Health Organization's List of Essential Medicines, the most effective and safe medicines needed in a health system. They are available as generic medication. In the United States a month of patches or gum is between 100 and 200 USD while the other forms are more expensive.

Medical uses

Nicotine replacement therapy, in the form of gum, patches, nasal spray, inhaler and lozenges all improve the ability of people trying to quit tobacco products. Studies have shown that nicotine replacement therapy is equally as effective as medications such as bupropion, in helping people quit smoking for at least 6 months. Studies have also shown that each form of nicotine replacement therapy, including nicotine gum, patches, nasal spray, inhalers, and lozenges have similar success rates in terms of helping people stop smoking. However, the likelihood that someone will stick to a certain treatment varied, with compliance being the highest with nicotine patches, followed by nicotine gum, inhalers, and nasal sprays. It is important to note that using a few different nicotine replacement methods in combination may improve one's success rates in stopping tobacco use. Additionally, using nicotine replacement with counseling has been proven to improve tobacco abstinence rates.

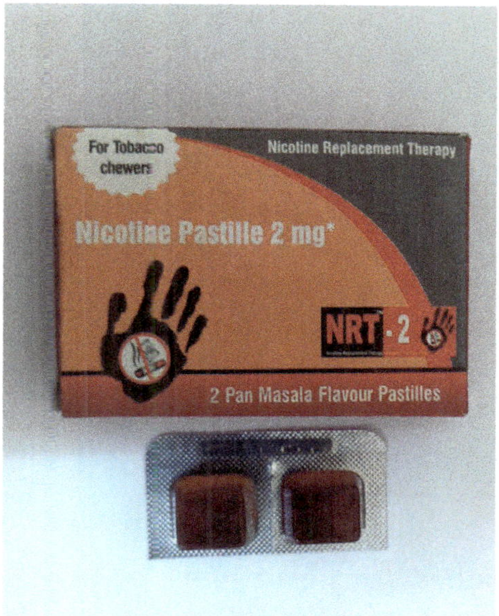

Nicotine pastilles

Nicotine replacement products are most beneficial for heavy smokers who smoke more than 15 cigarettes per day. There are not enough studies to show that NRT helps those who smoke fewer than 10 cigarettes per day.

Side Effects

While there is no evidence that NRT can increase the risk of heart attacks, individuals with pre-existing cardiovascular conditions or recent heart attacks should consult a physician before initiating NRT.

If you are under 18 years of age, you should consult your physician before starting NRT.

Nicotine exposure during pregnancy can result in attention deficit hyperactivity disorder (ADHD) and learning disabilities in the child. It also puts the child at risk for nicotine addiction in the future. Thus, pregnant women and those who are breastfeeding should also consult a physician before initiating NRT. The gum, lozenge, and nasal spray are pregnancy category C. The transdermal patch is pregnancy category D. The transdermal patch is considered less safe for the fetus because it delivers continuous nicotine exposure as opposed to the gum or lozenge, which delivers intermittent and thus lower nicotine exposure.

Limited evidence exists regarding long-term NRT use, and concerns exist that long-term NRT use could raise cancer risk, due in part to the generation of carcinogens.

Mechanism of Action

Nicotine replacement products vary in the time it takes for the nicotine to enter the body and the total time nicotine stays in the body.

Nicotine patches are applied to the skin and continuously administer a stable dose of nicotine slowly over 16–24 hours. Nicotine gum, nicotine sprays, nicotine sublingual tablets, and nicotine lozenges administer nicotine orally with quicker nicotine uptake into the body, but lasting a shorter amount of time. Nicotine inhalers are metered-dose inhalers that administer nicotine through the lungs and mucous membranes of the throat quickly, but lasting a short amount of time. For example, blood nicotine levels are the highest 5–10 minutes after using the nicotine nasal spray, 20 minutes after using a nicotine inhaler or chewing nicotine gum, and 2–4 hours after using a nicotine patch.

Society and Culture

Economics

In the United States a month of patches or gum is between 100 and 200 USD while the other forms are more expensive; in the UK lozenges are the cheapest. In the United States a month of patches is about 170 USD.

Exempted Populations

Evaluation of NRT in real-world studies produces more modest outcomes than efficacy studies conducted by the industry-funded trials. The National Health Service (NHS) in England has a smoking cessation service based on pharmacotherapy in combination with counseling support. An Action on Smoking and Health (UK) (ASH) report claims that the average cost per life year gained for every smoker successfully treated by these services is less than £1,000 (below the NICE guidelines of £20,000 per QALY (quality-adjusted life year). However, the investment in NHS stop smoking services is relatively low. A comparison with treatment costs for illicit drug users shows that £585 million is committed for 350,000 problem drug users compared to £56 million for 9 million users of tobacco. This is £6.20 for each smoker, compared to £1,670 per illegal drug user.

The claims for high efficacy and cost-effectiveness of NRT have not been substantiated in real-world effectiveness studies. Pierce and Gilpin (2002) stated their conclusion as follows: "Since becoming available over the counter, NRT appears no longer effective in increasing long-term successful cessation" . Efficacy studies, which are conducted using randomized controlled trials, do not transfer very well to real-world effectiveness. Bauld, Bell, McCullough, Richardson and Greaves (2009) reviewed 20 studies on the effectiveness of intensive NHS treatments for smoking cessation published between 1990 and 2007. Quit rates showed a dramatic decrease between 4-weeks and one year. A quit rate of 53% at four weeks fell to only 15% at 1 year. Younger smokers, females, pregnant smokers and more deprived smokers had lower quit rates than other groups.

In 2015, NRT sales fell for the first time since 2008 while sales for e-cigarettes continued to increase at a substantial rate. This had led to speculation that UK smokers are trying to quit with e-cigarettes rather than traditional, pharma-backed NRT methods.

Formulations

The United States Public Health Service lists seven agents for the stopping of tobacco, which include 5 nicotine replacement treatments (nicotine patches, gum, lozenges, inhalers, and nasal sprays) and 2 oral medications (bupropion and varenicline). Other NRT options are available, including nicotine mouth sprays and sublingual tablets.

Trade names include Nicotex, Nicorette, Nicoderm, Nicogum, Nicotinell, Thrive and Commit Lozenge.

Other Forms

Snus and nasal snuff also allow for nicotine administration outside of tobacco smoking, but do cause negative health effects.

E-cigarettes are often, although not always, designed to look and feel like cigarettes. They have been marketed as less harmful alternatives to cigarettes, but very few are as yet approved as NRTs in any jurisdiction. Some electronic cigarettes have coarsely adjustable nicotine levels. Some healthcare groups have hesitated to recommend e-cigarettes for quitting smoking, because of limited evidence of effectiveness and safety.

The U.S. Food and Drug Administration (FDA) has a list of additional tobacco products they are seeking to regulate, including electronic cigarettes. The evidence suggests that the FDA accepted products such as a nicotine inhaler may be a safer way to give nicotine than e-cigarettes.

Nicotine Patch

A nicotine patch is a transdermal patch that releases nicotine into the body through the skin. It is used as an aid in nicotine replacement therapy (NRT), a process for smoking cessation.

Medical Uses

Dozens of clinical trials have shown that the patch approximately doubles success rates over placebo treatment. Placebo tests show a 5.9% success rate, in comparison to the 7.2% blind active tests, and the 10.8% open tests.

Side Effects

Analysis of nicotine patches has shown that they contain tobacco-specific nitrosamines (TSNAs), known cancer-causing agents, in quantities of up to 173 mg per patch.

History

The first study of the pharmacokinetics of a transdermal nicotine patch in humans was published in 1984 by Jed E. Rose, Ph.D., Murray E. Jarvik, M.D., Ph.D. and K. Daniel Rose, and was followed by publication by Rose et al. (1985) of results of a study of smokers showing that a transdermal nicotine patch reduced craving for cigarettes. Frank Etscorn Ph.D. filed a patent in the United States on January the 23rd 1985 and was issued the patent on July 1, 1986. The University of California filed a competing patent application nearly 3 years after Etscorn's filing on February the 19th, 1988, which was granted on May 1, 1990. Subsequently, the U.S. Patent Office declared an interference action and, after a thorough review of conception, reduction to practice and patent filing dates, issued on September 29, 1993 a priority decision in favor of the Rose et al. patent.

Research

Nicotine patches are under study to help relieve the symptoms of post-surgical pain and treat early dementia.

Studies are being conducted about the use of transdermal nicotine patches to treat anxiety, depression, and inattentiveness in subjects with ADHD.

Transdermal nicotine patches can be used to relieve ulcerative colitis symptoms. However, this is not the case with Crohn's disease, a similar health condition, where smoking and nicotine intake in general worsen the disease's effects.

Varenicline

Varenicline (trade name Chantix and Champix usually in the form of varenicline tartrate), is a prescription medication used to treat nicotine addiction. Varenicline is a nicotinic receptor partial agonist—it stimulates nicotine receptors more weakly than nicotine itself does. In this respect it is similar to cytisine and different from the nicotinic antagonist, bupropion, and nicotine replacement therapies (NRTs) like nicotine patches and nicotine gum. As a partial agonist it both reduces cravings for and decreases the pleasurable effects of cigarettes and other tobacco products. Through these mechanisms it can assist some patients to quit smoking.

Medical uses

Varenicline is used for smoking cessation. In a 2009 meta-analysis varenicline was found to be more effective than bupropion (odds ratio 1.40) and NRTs (odds ratio 1.56).

A 2013 Cochrane overview and network meta-analysis concluded that varenicline is the most effective medication for tobacco cessation and that smokers were nearly three times more likely to quit on varenicline than with placebo treatment. Varenicline was more efficacious than bupropion or NRT and as effective as combination NRT for tobacco smoking cessation.

The United States' Food and Drug Administration (US FDA) has approved the use of varenicline for up to twelve weeks. If smoking cessation has been achieved it may be continued for another twelve weeks.

Varenicline has not been tested in those under 18 years old or pregnant women and therefore is not recommended for use by these groups. Varenicline is considered a class C pregnancy drug, as animal studies have shown no increased risk of congenital anomalies, however, no data from human studies is available. An observational study is currently being conducted assessing for malformations related to varenicline exposure, but has no results yet. An alternate drug is preferred for smoking cessation during breastfeeding due to lack of information and based on the animal studies on nicotine.

Side Effects

Mild nausea is the most common side effect and is seen in approximately 30% of people taking varenicline though this rarely (<3%) results in discontinuation of the medication. Other less common side effects include headache, difficulty sleeping, and nightmares. Rare side effects reported by people taking varenicline compared to placebo include change in taste, vomiting, abdominal pain, flatulence, and constipation. In a recent meta-analysis paper by Leung *et al.*, it has been estimated that for every five subjects taking varenicline at maintenance doses, there will be an event of nausea, and for every 24 and 35 treated subjects, there will be an event of constipation and flatulence respectively. Gastrointestinal side-effects lead to discontinuation of the drug in 2% to 8% of people using varenicline. Incidence of nausea is dose-dependent: incidence of nausea was higher in people taking a larger dose (30%) versus placebo (10%) as compared to people taking a smaller dose (16%) versus placebo (11%).

Depression and Suicide

A 2014 systematic review did not find evidence of an increased suicide risk. Other analyses have reached the same conclusion and found no increased risk of neuropsychiatric side effects with varenicline. No evidence for increased risks of cardiovascular events, depression, or self-harm with varenicline versus nicotine replacement therapy has been found in one post-marketing surveillance study.

In 2007, the US FDA had announced it had received post-marketing reports of thoughts of suicide and occasional suicidal behavior, erratic behavior, and drowsiness among people using varenicline for smoking cessation. In 2009, the US FDA required varenicline to carry a boxed warning that the drug should be stopped if any of these symptoms are experienced. In 2016 the FDA removed the black box warning. People are still advised to stop the medication if they "notice any side effects on mood, behavior, or thinking."

Cardiovascular Disease

In June 2011, the US FDA issued a safety announcement that varenicline may be associated with "a small, increased risk of certain cardiovascular adverse events in people who have cardiovascular disease."

A prior 2011 review had found increased risk of cardiovascular events compared with placebo. Expert commentary in the same journal raised doubts about the methodology of the review, concerns which were echoed by the European Medicines Agency and subsequent reviews. Of specific concern were "the low number of events seen, the types of events counted, the higher drop-out rate in people receiving placebo, the lack of information on the timing of events, and the exclusion of studies in which no-one had an event."

In contrast, multiple recent systematic reviews and meta-analyses have found no increase in overall or serious adverse cardiovascular events (including for individuals at risk of developing cardiovascular disease) associated with varenicline use.

Mechanism of Action

Varenicline displays full agonism on α_7 nicotinic acetylcholine receptors and is a partial agonist on the $\alpha_4\beta_2$, $\alpha_3\beta_4$, and $\alpha_6\beta_2$ subtypes. In addition, it is a weak agonist on the $\alpha_3\beta_2$ containing receptors.

Varenicline's partial agonism on the $\alpha_4\beta_2$ receptors rather than nicotine's full agonism produces less effect of dopamine release than nicotine's. This $\alpha_4\beta_2$ competitive binding reduces the ability of nicotine to bind and stimulate the mesolimbic dopamine system - similar to the method of action of buprenorphine in the treatment of opioid addiction.

Pharmacokinetics

Most of the active compound is excreted by the kidneys (92–93%). A small proportion is glucuronidated, oxidised, *N*-formylated or conjugated to a hexose. The elimination half-life is about 24 hours.

History

Use of Cytisus plant as a smoking substitute during World War II led to use as a cessation aid in eastern Europe and extraction of cytisine. Cytisine analogs led to varenicline at Pfizer.

Varenicline received a "priority review" by the US FDA in February 2006, shortening the usual 10-month review period to 6 months because of its demonstrated effectiveness in clinical trials and perceived lack of safety issues. The agency's approval of the drug came on May 11, 2006. On August 1, 2006, varenicline was made available for sale in the United States and on September 29, 2006, was approved for sale in the European Union.

Coding (Therapy)

Coding (also known as the Dovzhenko method) is a catch-all term for various Russian alternative therapeutic methods used to treat addictions, in which the therapist attempts to scare patients into abstinence from a substance they are addicted to by convincing them that they will be harmed or killed if they use it again. Each method involves the therapist pretending to insert a "code" into patients' brains that will ostensibly provoke a strong adverse reaction should it come into contact with the addictive substance. The methods use a combination of theatrics, hypnosis, placebos, and drugs with temporary adverse effects to instill the erroneous beliefs. Therapists may pretend to "code" patients for a fixed length of time, such as five years.

Coding was created by Alexander Dovzhenko, a psychiatrist in the former Soviet Union. It has been widely used to treat alcohol addiction in Russia, but 16 percent of Russian narcologists also report using it in their practices.

Methods

In the case of alcohol addiction, the procedure may be carried out with a drug that temporarily affects the respiratory system when mixed with alcohol, administered under hypnosis. The therapist gives patients the drug, then allows them a small amount of alcohol, which triggers an adverse reaction and makes them erroneously believe that the therapy has had a long-term effect. Another method involves the therapist giving patients hypnotic suggestions during a head massage, with the message that alcohol will cause blindness or paralysis.

In one method, the therapist numbs patients' mouths with local anaesthetic, then places electrodes with a very weak current into their mouths. This is to make patients believe that the "nerve points" in their mouth are being "manipulated" and that it is no longer safe for them to drink alcohol. A further method involves the therapist using a special helmet to persuade patients that the therapist's suggestions are controlling their minds. Typically, therapists will also make patients sign a disclaimer, supposedly absolving the therapist of any responsibility should the patient use the addictive substance and suffer ill effects or die.

Contingency Management

Contingency management (CM) is most-widely used in the field of substance abuse, often implemented as part of clinical behavior analysis. CM refers to the application of the three-term contingency (or operant conditioning), which uses stimulus control and positive reinforcement to change behavior. Patients' behaviors are rewarded (or, less often, punished); generally, adherence to or failure to adhere to program rules and regulations or their treatment plan. CM derives from the science of applied behavior analysis (ABA), and by most evaluations, its procedures produces one of the largest effect sizes out of all mental health and educational interventions.

Token Economies

One form of contingency management is the token economy system. Token systems can be used in an individual or group format. Token systems have been shown to be successful with a diverse array of populations including those suffering from addiction, those with special needs, and delinquents. However, recent research questions the use of token systems with very young children. The exception to the last would be the treatment of stuttering. The goal of such systems is to gradually thin out and to help the person begin to access the natural community of reinforcement (the reinforcement typically received in the world for performing the behavior).

Walker (1990) presents an overview of token systems and combining such procedures with other interventions in the classroom. He relates the comprehensiveness of token systems to the child's level of difficulty.

Voucher Programs and Related Applications in Addiction Treatment

Another form of contingency management is voucher programs. In voucher-based contingency management patients earn vouchers exchangeable for retail items contingent upon objectively verified abstinence from recent drug use or compliance with other behavior-change targets. This particular form of contingency management was introduced in the early 1990s as a treatment for cocaine dependence. The approach is the most reliably effective method for producing cocaine abstinence in controlled clinical trials.

Medication take-home privileges is another form of contingency management frequently used in methadone maintenance treatment. Patients are permitted to "earn" take-home doses of their methadone in exchange for increasing, decreasing, or ceasing certain behaviors. For example, a patient may be given one take-home dose per week after submitting negative drug screens (generally via urine testing) for three months. (It is worth noting that take home-doses (or "bottles") are seen as desirable rewards because they allow patients to come to the clinic less often to obtain their medication).

Based in applied behavior analysis (ABA), contingency management includes techniques such as choice, shaping, time-out, making contracts between the therapist and patient, and token economy.

Contingent vouchers are also used to cease smoking addictions. One study claims that addicts with substance use disorders can receive help with their addiction through the use of voucher-based treatment for smoking. In addition, nicotine replacement (NRT) can help with addiction combined with the vouchers.

Level Systems

Level systems are often employed as a form of contingency management system. Level systems are designed such that once one level is achieved, then the person earns all the privileges for that level and the levels lower than it.

Effectiveness in Addiction Programs

A recent meta-analysis of contingency management in drug programs showed that it has a large effect. These contingencies are delivered based on abstinence and attendance goals and can take the form of vouchers, the opportunity to win prizes, or privileges. They have been used with single problem addictions as well as dual diagnoses and homeless. Overall contingency management has been found to be an effective and cost efficient addition to drug treatment.

In contrast to these findings in a recent study, the researchers found out that Nicotine replacement treatment only improved the effects of contingent vouchers on short-term smoking abstinence. However, in the long term the effects of contingent vouchers had no impact on tobacco resistance.

Organizations

Many organizations exists for board certified behavior analysts using contingency management around the world.

Community Reinforcement Approach and Family Training

Community reinforcement approach and family training (CRAFT) is a behavior therapy approach for treating addiction. The original community reinforcement approach (CRA) developed by Nate Azrin in the 1970s uses operant conditioning to help people learn to reduce the power of their addictions and enjoy healthy life. CRAFT combines CRA with family training, which equips family and friends with supportive techniques to encourage their loved ones to begin and continue treatment, and provides defenses against addiction's damaging effects on loved ones.

The *community reinforcement approach* (CRA) was "originally developed for individuals with alcohol use disorders, [and] has been successfully employed to treat a variety of substance use disorders for more than 35 years. Based on operant conditioning [a type of learning], CRA helps people rearrange their lifestyles so that healthy, drug-free living becomes rewarding and thereby competes with alcohol and drug use."

"CRA is a time-limited treatment." "In time-limited therapy, a set number of sessions (for example, 16 sessions) or time limit (for example, one year) is decided upon either at the very beginning of therapy or within the early stages of therapy."

Community reinforcement and family training (CRAFT) is CRA that "works through family member." It "is designed to increase the odds of the substance user who is refusing treatment to enter treatment, as well as improve the lives of the concerned family members. CRAFT "teaches the use of healthy rewards to encourage positive behaviors. Plus, it focuses on helping both the substance user and the family."

Adolescent Community Reinforcement Approach (A-CRA) is CRA that "targets adolescents with substance use problems and their caregivers."

Description

Community Reinforcement Approach and Family Training (CRAFT) is a motivational model of family therapy. It is reward-based—based on positive reinforcement. CRAFT is aimed at the families and friends of treatment-refusing individuals who have a substance abuse problem. "CRAFT works to affect [(influence)] the substance users' behavior by changing the way the family interacts with them."

In the model, the following terms are used:

- *Identified Patient* (IP) - the individual with the substance abuse problem that is refusing treatment, and

- *Concerned Significant Others* (CSOs) - the relevant family and friends of the IP.

"CRAFT grew out of the understanding that although individuals who truly need help with substance use problems often are strongly opposed to treatment. On the other hand, the concerned significant others (CSOs) of the substance abuser are commonly highly motivated to get help for them."

Three Goals

When a loved one is abusing substances and refusing to get help, CRAFT is designed to help families learn practical and effective ways to accomplish these three goals:

1. move their loved one toward treatment,
2. reduce their loved one's alcohol and drug use, and
3. simultaneously improve their own lives.

One experiment compared CRAFT against and Al-Anon and Nar-Anon facilitation therapy in their impact on the addict entering treatment and found concerned significant others who participated in Al-Anon and Nar-Anon facilitation therapy engaged 29.0% of addicts whereas those who went through CRAFT engaged 67.2%. Another study compared CRAFT, Al-Anon facilitation therapy designed to encourage involvement in the 12-step program, and a Johnson intervention and found that all of these approaches were associated with similar improvements in concerned significant other functioning and improvements in their relationship quality with the addict. However, the CRAFT approach was more effective in engaging initially unmotivated problem drinkers in treatment (64%) as compared with the Al-Anon (13%) and Johnson interventions (30%).

Family Influence

Robert J. Meyers, Ph.D. writes about the influence that concerned family members—called *Concerned Significant Others* (CSOs)—have in treatment of the substance user, and the benefits for themselves:

The Community Reinforcement Approach and Family Training (CRAFT) intervention method was developed with the belief that since family members can, and do make important contribution[s] in other areas of addiction treatment (i.e. family and couples therapy), that the CSO can play a powerful role in helping to engage the substance user who is in denial to submit to treatment. In addition, it is often the substance user who reports that family pressure or influence is the reason [they] sought treatment. Also, CSOs who attend the CRAFT program also benefit by becoming more independent and reducing their depression, anxiety and anger symptoms even if their loved one does not enter treatment.

CRA Procedures

The following CRA procedures and descriptions are from Meyers, Roozen, and Smith for the substance user:

1. Functional Analysis of Substance
    - explore the antecedents of a client's substance use
    - explore the positive and negative consequences of a client's substance use
2. Sobriety Sampling
    - a gentle movement toward long-term abstinence that begins with a client's agreement to sample a time-limited period of abstinence
3. CRA Treatment Plan
    - establish meaningful, objective goals in client-selected areas
    - establish highly specified methods for obtaining those goals
    - tools: Happiness Scale, and Goals of Counseling form
4. Behavior Skills Training
    - teach three basic skills through instruction and role-playing:
        1. Problem-solving
            - break overwhelming problems into smaller ones
            - address smaller problems
        2. Communication skills
            - a positive interaction style
        3. Drink/drug refusal training
            - identify high-risk situations
            - teach assertiveness
5. Job Skills Training
    - provide basic steps for obtaining and keeping a valued job
6. Social and Recreational Counseling
    - provide opportunities to sample new social and recreational activities

7. Relapse Prevention
   - teach clients how to identify high-risk situations
   - teach clients how to anticipate and cope with a relapse
8. Relationship Counseling
   - improve the interaction between the client and his or her partner

CRAFT Communication

With CRAFT, families/friends (CSOs) are trained in various strategies, including positive reinforcement, various communication skills and natural consequences. "One of the big pieces that has a lot of influence over all the other strategies is positive communication. "There are seven steps in the CRAFT model for implementing positive communication strategies."

1. Be Brief
2. Be Positive
3. Refer to Specific Behaviors
4. Label your Feelings
5. Offer an Understanding Statement - For example, "I appreciate that you have these concerns, [or] I understand that you really want to talk right now, and that this feels urgent, [or] I would love to be there for you."
6. Accept Partial Responsibility - This step "is really designed to decrease defensiveness on the part of your loved one. It's not about accepting responsibility for things you are not responsible for. [Rather, it's to] direct you towards the piece that you can own for yourself. [For example,] what you can take responsibility for are the ways that you communicate," etc.
7. Offer to help

"The overarching goals for the strategies for communicating are to help decrease defensiveness on the part of the loved one that you are speaking to, and increase the chances that your message is really going to be heard—so, increasing the ability that you have to really get across the message that you want." In fact, the title of Robert J. Meyers' and Brenda L. Wolfe's book based on CRAFT is, *Get Your Loved One Sober: Alternatives to Nagging, Pleading, and Threatening*.

"Consequences being in place is really important and helpful in terms of communicating your message, but it's also really important, maybe even moreso, to be consistent in following through with those consequences and rewards."

Al-Anon and CRAFT

According to the suggested prologue read at many Al-Anon meetings, Al-Anon holds that, "We believe alcoholism is a family illness and that changed attitudes can aid recovery.Al-Anon has but one purpose: to help families of alcoholics. We do this by practicing the Twelve Steps, by welcoming and giving comfort to families of alcoholics, and by giving understanding and encouragement to the alcoholic." Their suggested welcome clearly states that, "The family situation is bound to improve as we apply the Al-Anon ideas." Al-Anon believes that alcoholism is a family disease, and that as a result of trying, often for years, to cope with the substance abuse related behaviors of others, family members may become, "Irritable and unreasonable without knowing it". Because it is common for family members to exert significant energy on counter-productive interventions with loved ones, Al-Anon's pamphlet on detachment counsels that concerned significant others "detach with love"; this means,"Separating ourselves from the adverse effects of another person's alcoholism can be a means of detaching: this does not necessarily require physical separation. Detachment can help us look at our situations realistically and objectively." Counter-productive behaviors for family members and their substance abusers include the very behaviors that CRAFT seeks to remedy--yelling, screaming, pleading, engaging the alcoholic while he or she is using, manipulation and counter-manipulation, negativity, defensiveness and anger. The skills Al-Anon seeks to teach, according to their pamphlet on detachment, are:

"IN AL-ANON WE LEARN: • Not to suffer because of the actions or reactions of other people • Not to allow ourselves to be used or abused by others in the interest of another's recovery • Not to do for others what they can do for themselves • Not to manipulate situations so others will eat, go to bed, get up, pay bills, notdrink, or behave as we see fit • Not to cover up for another's mistakes or misdeeds • Not to create a crisis • Not to prevent a crisis if it is in the natural course of events

By learning to focus on ourselves, our attitudes and well-being improve. We allow the alcoholics in our lives to experience the consequences of their own actions."

Al-Anon does not currently adopt, hold, or promote the view that concerned significant others (CSOs) can with any certainty make a positive, direct, and active contribution to arrest compulsive drinking; Al-Anon does, however, say that by improving our own attitudes and offering support an encouragement to the alcoholic the "family situation is bound to improve". The premise of CRAFT is that deliberate, positive interactions can increase willingness and decrease resistance. Al-Anon recognizes that while increased willingness and decreased resistance may be a happy by-product of detaching from the adverse behaviors of alcoholics, there are no guarantees that this will occur. Al-Anon is a fellowship with a focus on helping families and friends, themselves, without promoting a direct intervention process for alcoholics. Because "no one ever graduates" from Al-Anon, it can be viewed as an open-ended program, not time-limited; it is available for concerned significant others as long as they may need it, and there are thousands of Al-Anon meetings around the country held on a weekly basis.

Al-Anon View

Regarding the CSO's relationship to alcoholism and sobriety, the view from the Al-Anon organization can be summarized:

1. *Powerlessness.* Al-Anon's First Step promotes a powerless view for families and friends, "We admitted we were powerless over alcohol—that our lives had become unmanageable."

2. *Disease view.* Al-Anon writes, "As the American Medical Association will attest, alcoholism is a disease." Al-Anon also states, "Although it can be arrested, alcoholism has no known cure."

3. *Three C's.* Al-Anon has a dictum called "the Three C's—I didn't cause alcoholism; I can't control it; and I can't cure it."

4. *Loving detachment.* Al-Anon "advocates 'loving detachment' from the substance abuser." It is important to note that this is often confused with rejecting or socially isolating the alcoholic; in fact, it simply means that we are responsible for our own actions alone, not the actions of and choices of anyone else. This notion of personal responsibility is particularly important for those who may blame themselves when they are subjected to the domestic violence, emotional harm, financial malfeasance and insecurity, or a myriad of other painful and troubling outcomes often associated with having an substance abuser in the family. It does not mean that we cease to love, care for, encourage, communicate with, or otherwise cease positive interactions with a loved one unless the concerned significant other makes a conscious, thoughtful decision to do so.

    - *Family illness.* Al-Anon writes, "Alcoholism is a family disease," and "we believe alcoholism is a family illness and that changed attitudes can aid recovery."

Regarding alcoholics, the Al-Anon-recommended approach for CSOs (families/friends) is "detachment with love" and "giving understanding and encouragement to the alcoholic."

No Direct Impact

As far as the CSOs having a direct and positive impact on another's sobriety, Al-Anon asks itself:

"But surely," we argue, "sobriety is desirable, and there must be something we can do to help! There has to be something we can say that will make a difference, or some sort of help or support or information we can provide that will convince our alcoholic loved ones to get the help they need or to make sure they continue on the path to recovery!"

Al-Anon answers:

Alcoholism is a disease. Would the right word stop the spread of cancer or make chemotherapy more effective? Would our help, good looks, higher income, or cleaner house overcome the progression of Alzheimer's Disease? Our compassion and support might make a loved one's struggle with illness easier to bear, but it is simply not within our power to cure someone else's disease. We are powerless over another's alcoholism.

This answer has these three characteristics:

1. *Absolute outcomes.* Regarding *help*, their answer tends toward complete and total outcomes, such as the ability for someone to *convince, cure* or *overcome* someone else's alcoholism, or that they could guarantee *(make sure)* that someone continues on the path to recovery. Although this answer may help dispel the notion that someone has permanent, guaranteed power over another's sobriety, it does not answer the question that someone could provide *any* measure of direct help or support toward someone else's sobriety or treatment of someone else's addiction.

2. *Incomplete analogies.* They write that *the right word* can neither make chemotherapy—a bio-chemical process—more effective nor *stop* cancer. However, their answer does not address the *help* or *support* or *information* that could make cancer treatment more effective or that could have a positive impact against cancer.

3. *Medical opinion.* Modern contrary assessments exist that alcohol (and drug) addiction are *not* (progressive, incurable) diseases, coming from Dr. Gene Heyman and others. In 1960, Bill Wilson—the co-founder of A.A. (his wife Lois was co-founder of Al-Anon)—called alcoholism a *malady or illness* and did not view it as a disease. The diagnostic assessment of alcoholism in someone can include an assessment of co-morbidity, mental illness, and domestic violence.

CRAFT View

The work of Robert Meyers' CRAFT Community Reinforcement Approach and Family Training program differs significantly from Al-Anon in that it is a behavioral program which advocates that the CSO *[Concerned Significant Other]* can have a positive impact on the substance abuser. The CRAFT program has been demonstrated in Meyers' research to be more effective than the Vernon Johnson type intervention or Al-Anon, with less negative side-effects and better outcomes, whether or not the substance abuser enters treatment.

The CRAFT program uses a variety of interventions based on functional assessment including a module to prevent domestic violence.

Intervention and CRAFT

"There are questions about the long-term effectiveness of interventions for those addicted to drugs or alcohol. A study examining addicts who had undergone a standard intervention (called the Johnson Intervention) found that they had a higher relapse rate than any other method of referral to outpatient Alcohol and Other Drug treatment".

Smith, Campos-Melady and Meyers describe the Johnson Institute intervention as a "surprise party" that is uncomfortable for many CSOs (families/friends):

The Al-Anon approach's emphasis upon detaching from the substance abuser is unappealing to many CSOs. On the other end of the spectrum is the Johnson Institute Intervention: a "surprise party" in which the IP is confronted by family members and a therapist with the objective of getting the IP to enter treatment. When the intervention is actually carried out, it often results in a high rate of engagement in treatment, and yet only a small number of CSOs who begin the program ever follow through with the intervention (Liepman, Nirenberg, & Begin, 1989; Miller et al., 1999), and many report feeling uncomfortable with its confrontational nature (Barber & Gilbertson, 1997).

Research suggests that CRAFT has had much more success than the Johnson Intervention method or Al-Anon/Alateen as far as engaging loved ones in treatment.

Research and Outcomes

CRA

The community reinforcement approach has considerable research supporting it as effective. Community reinforcement has both efficacy and effectiveness data. Started in the 1970s, community reinforcement approach is a comprehensive operant program built on a functional assessment of a client's drinking behavior and the use of positive reinforcement and contingency management for non-drinking. When combined with disulfiram (an aversive procedure) community reinforcement showed remarkable effects. One component of the program that appears to be particularly strong is the non-drinking club. Applications of community reinforcement to public policy has become the recent focus of this approach.

Outpatient

"The Community Reinforcement Approach has been found to be extremely effective in outpatient settings as well. In one study, clients treated with CRA and the disulfiram compliance component were abstinent an average of 97% of the days during the last month of the 6-month followup, whereas clients treated with a combination of a 12-step program and the CRA disulfiram compliance training were abstinent an average of 74% of the days. For those clients who received a 12-step program and a prescription for disulfiram, an average of only 45% of the comparable days were abstinent (Azrin, Sisson, Meyers, & Godley, 1982)."

CRAFT (and Al-Anon, Intervention, etc.)

An offshoot of the community reinforcement approach is the community reinforcement approach and family training. This program is designed to help family members of substance abusers feel empowered to engage in treatment. Community reinforcement approach and family training (CRAFT) has helped family members to get their loved ones into treatment. The rates of success have varied somewhat by study but seem to cluster around 70%. CRAFT is one of the only family-aimed treatments with proven results for getting people with drug or alcohol problems into treatment. The program uses a variety of interventions based on functional assessment including a module to prevent domestic violence. Partners are trained to use positive reinforcement, various communication skills and natural consequences.

Alcohol Abusers Intervention

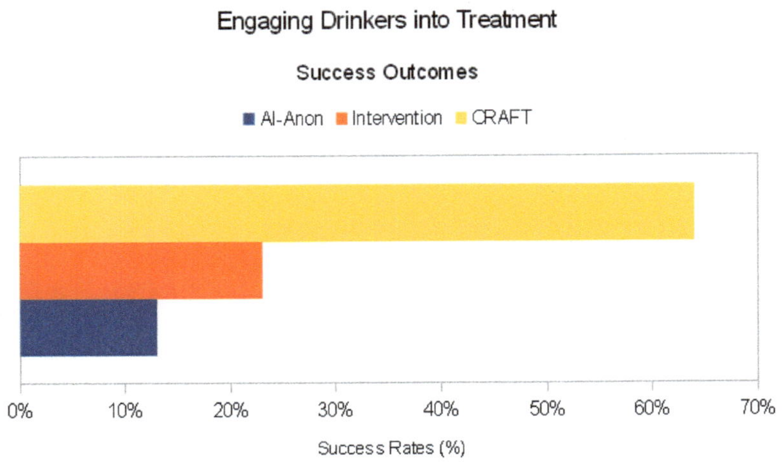

Results and Safety

From an article on the American Psychology Association (APA) website about the success of CRAFT in substance abuse treatment and intervention, these are the success outcomes for engaging drinkers into treatment:

1. 64% - CRAFT
2. 23% - Johnson Intervention
3. 13% - Al-Anon

From the article:

Sisson and Azrin (1986) recruited 12 adult women with an alcoholic husband, brother, or father and randomly assigned them either to an early version of CRAFT or to a traditional intervention. Results indicated that CRAFT was considerably more successful in getting the persons with substance abuse into treatment and reducing their alcohol consumption in comparison to the Al-Anon group. Miller et al. (1999) conducted a controlled comparison of CRAFT, the Johnson Intervention, and Al-Anon facilitation (TSF) that randomized 130 caregivers of problem drinkers to receive 12 hours of contact in one of the three conditions. CRAFT and TSF had better retention than the Johnson Intervention. Consistent with previous studies, participants tended to drop out of the latter intervention in order to avoid the family confrontation with the drinker. The CRAFT intervention also engaged substantially more drinkers into treatment (64% vs 23% Johnson and 13% TSF).

Drug Abusers Intervention

From the same article on the American Psychology Association (APA) website about the success of CRAFT in substance abuse treatment and intervention, these are the success outcomes for persons abusing drugs to enter treatment (the success outcomes were nearly the same as the alcohol abuse outcomes):

1. 64% - CRAFT
2. 17% - Caregivers' Twelve-step Self-help Group (TSG)

From the article:

Kirby et al. (1999) randomly assigned 32 caregivers of drug users to CRAFT or a 12-step self-help group (TSG). Caregivers who were assigned to CRAFT attended more sessions than those in TSG and were more likely to complete a full course of counseling during which the persons abusing drugs were far more likely to enter treatment (64% vs 17%). Reductions in drug use occurred during the study, but there was no group x time interaction. Meyers et al. (2002) replicated and extended those findings with drug users with similar positive effects on engagement of the drug abusing family members in treatment.

Note: When the articles states "there was no group x time interaction," it simply means the CRAFT outcome (64%) and the TSF outcome (17%) remained the same over time, even though there was a reduction in drug use during the study.

Parallel Study

"In a parallel study sponsored by the National Institute on Drug Abuse that focused on abusers of other drugs, family members receiving CRAFT successfully engaged 74 percent of initially unmotivated drug users in treatment (Meyers et al. 1999)."

History

The most influential behaviorist of all times, B. F. Skinner, largely considered punishment to be an ineffective method for modifying human behavior (Skinner 1974). Thus it was no surprise that, many years later, research discovered that substance use disorder treatments based on confrontation were largely ineffective in decreasing the use of alcohol and other substances (Miller and Wilbourne 2002, Miller et al. 1998). Nate Azrin already was convinced of this back in the early 1970s, when he designed an innovative treatment for alcohol problems: the Community Reinforcement Approach (CRA). Azrin believed that it was necessary to alter the environment in which people with alcohol problems live so that they received strong reinforcement for sober behavior from their community, including family, work, and friends. As part of this strategy, the program emphasizes helping clients discover new, enjoyable activities that do not revolve around alcohol, and teaching them the skills necessary for participating in those activities.

The Origin of CRAFT

Drs. Robert J. Meyers and Jane Ellen Smith of the University of New Mexico developed the CRAFT program to teach families how to impact their loved one while avoiding both detachment and confrontation, the respective strategies of Al-Anon (a 12-Step based approach), and traditional (Johnson Institute-style) interventions in which the substance user is confronted by family members and friends during a surprise meeting. While all three approaches have been found to improve family members' functioning and relationship satisfaction, CRAFT has proven to be significantly more effective in engaging loved ones in comparison to the Johnson Institute Intervention or Al-Anon/Nar-Anon facilitation therapy.

2009

Up to 2009, CRAFT and CRA programs were not widespread amongst addiction counselors. Instead, many addiction counselors were tied to a twelve-step model that had much less research support. Recent trends by the National Institute on Drug Abuse (NIDA) have been to help deploy these intervention techniques. In 2007, CRAFT was being used in 25 clinics in the United States.

Professional Organizations

Association for Behavior Analysis International

The Association for Behavior Analysis International (ABAI) has a special interest group in clinical behavior analysis and behavioral counseling ABA:I. The association is developing a special interest group for behavioral pharmacology and addictions. The association serves as the core intellectual home for behavior analysts. The ABAI sponsors two conferences per year—one in the U.S., and one internationally.

Association for Behavioral and Cognitive Therapies

The Association for Behavioral and Cognitive Therapies (ABCT) also has an interest group in behavior analysis, which focuses on clinical behavior analysis. In addition, ABCT has a special interest group on addictions.

References

- C.R. Ganellin; David J. Triggle (21 November 1996). Dictionary of Pharmacological Agents. CRC Press. pp. 1396–. ISBN 978-0-412-46630-4
- "FDA Approves New Drug for Treatment of Alcoholism". FDA Talk Paper. Food and Drug Administration. 2004-07-29. Archived from the original on 2008-01-17. Retrieved 2009-08-15
- Berman, S; Noble, EP (1993). "Childhood antecedents of substance misuse". Current Opinion in Psychiatry. 6 (3): 382–7. doi:10.1097/00001504-199306000-00012
- Mason, BJ (2001). "Treatment of alcohol-dependent outpatients with acamprosate: a clinical review.". The Journal of Clinical Psychiatry. 62 Suppl 20: 42–8. PMID 11584875
- Daphne Simeon; Jeffrey Abugel (10 October 2008). Feeling Unreal: Depersonalization Disorder and the Loss of the Self. Oxford University Press. pp. 166–. ISBN 978-0-19-976635-2
- Therapeutic Goods Administration. "Australian Register of Therapeutic Goods Medicines" (Online database of approved medicines). Retrieved 2009-03-22
- Larimer, Robert C. (September 13, 1952). "Treatment of Alcoholism with Antabuse". Journal of the American Medical Association. 150 (2): 79. doi:10.1001/jama.1952.03680020013004. Retrieved 2016-03-11
- Musto, David F. (1999). The American Disease: Origins of Narcotic Control (3rd ed.). Oxford University Press. p. 76. ISBN 0195125096
- Novella, Steven (5 May 2010). "Low Dose Naltrexone – Bogus or Cutting Edge Science?". Science-Based Medicine. Retrieved 5 July 2011
- Daynes, G; Gillman MA (1994). "Psychotropic analgesic nitrous oxide prevents craving after withdrawal from alcohol, cannabis and tobacco". Int J Neurosci. 76 (1-2): 13–16. doi:10.3109/00207459408985987
- Smith, KD; Scott, MA; Ketterman, E; Smith, PO (April 2005). "Clinical inquiries. What interventions can help patients stop using chewing tobacco?". The Journal of family practice. 54 (4): 368–9. PMID 15833231
- Beck, Aaron T.; Wright, Fred D.; Newman, Cory F.; Liese, Bruce S. (16 January 2001). "Ch 11: Focus on Beliefs". Cognitive Therapy of Substance Abuse. Guilford Press. pp. 169–186. ISBN 978-1-57230-659-2
- "Addiction & Alcohol Rehab, Alcohol Detox, Drug Rehabilitation In Peterborough, UK.". Addiction Rehab Peterborough. Retrieved 10 November 2016
- Rigotti, NA (Feb 2002). "Clinical practice. Treatment of tobacco use and dependence.". The New England Journal of Medicine. 346 (7): 506–12. PMID 11844853. doi:10.1056/nejmcp012279
- Evans, Katie; Sullivan, Michael J. (1 March 2001). Dual Diagnosis: Counseling the Mentally Ill Substance Abuser (2nd ed.). Guilford Press. pp. 75–76. ISBN 978-1-57230-446-8

- Renshaw, Amy. "The Real Story Behind the Nicotine Patch and Smoking Cessation". vanderbilt. edu. Vanderbilt University. Retrieved 25 November 2013
- Bostwick, J. Michael; Bucci, Jeffrey A. (2008). "Internet Sex Addiction Treated with Naltrexone". Mayo Clinic Proceedings. 83 (2): 226–30. PMID 18241634. doi:10.4065/83.2.226
- Birnbrauer, J.S., Wolf, M.M., Kidder, J.D., & Tague, C.E. (1965). "Classroom behavior of retarded pupils with token reinforcement". Journal of Experimental Child Psychology, 2, 219–235
- Hamilton, Richart (2015). Tarascon Pocket Pharmacopoeia 2015 Deluxe Lab-Coat Edition. Jones & Bartlett Learning. p. 441. ISBN 9781284057560
- Kuehn BM (2006). "FDA speeds smoking cessation drug review". JAMA. 295 (6): 614–614. PMID 16467225. doi:10.1001/jama.295.6.614

Permissions

All chapters in this book are published with permission under the Creative Commons Attribution Share Alike License or equivalent. Every chapter published in this book has been scrutinized by our experts. Their significance has been extensively debated. The topics covered herein carry significant information for a comprehensive understanding. They may even be implemented as practical applications or may be referred to as a beginning point for further studies.

We would like to thank the editorial team for lending their expertise to make the book truly unique. They have played a crucial role in the development of this book. Without their invaluable contributions this book wouldn't have been possible. They have made vital efforts to compile up to date information on the varied aspects of this subject to make this book a valuable addition to the collection of many professionals and students.

This book was conceptualized with the vision of imparting up-to-date and integrated information in this field. To ensure the same, a matchless editorial board was set up. Every individual on the board went through rigorous rounds of assessment to prove their worth. After which they invested a large part of their time researching and compiling the most relevant data for our readers.

The editorial board has been involved in producing this book since its inception. They have spent rigorous hours researching and exploring the diverse topics which have resulted in the successful publishing of this book. They have passed on their knowledge of decades through this book. To expedite this challenging task, the publisher supported the team at every step. A small team of assistant editors was also appointed to further simplify the editing procedure and attain best results for the readers.

Apart from the editorial board, the designing team has also invested a significant amount of their time in understanding the subject and creating the most relevant covers. They scrutinized every image to scout for the most suitable representation of the subject and create an appropriate cover for the book.

The publishing team has been an ardent support to the editorial, designing and production team. Their endless efforts to recruit the best for this project, has resulted in the accomplishment of this book. They are a veteran in the field of academics and their pool of knowledge is as vast as their experience in printing. Their expertise and guidance has proved useful at every step. Their uncompromising quality standards have made this book an exceptional effort. Their encouragement from time to time has been an inspiration for everyone.

The publisher and the editorial board hope that this book will prove to be a valuable piece of knowledge for students, practitioners and scholars across the globe.

Index

A

Addiction Medicine, 15, 87, 92, 153, 167-168

Addiction Psychology, 151-152, 154-155, 157

Addiction Severity Index, 135, 153

Addiction Treatment, 40, 87, 153, 155, 157, 164, 179, 185, 194, 208, 211

Addiction Vulnerability, 160-162

Adrenal Medulla, 20, 27

Alcohol Addiction, 11, 45, 184, 207

Alcohol Withdrawal, 12, 37, 45-48, 52, 107, 168, 170

Alcoholism, 2-3, 16-17, 31-33, 35-40, 42-50, 52, 78, 89, 100, 106, 109, 134, 150, 152-153, 157, 166, 171-172, 175, 182, 185-186, 193-194, 214-216, 221

American Psychological Association, 150, 154-155, 165

Amphetamine, 2, 5-6, 9, 13, 17, 52-72, 90, 101, 105, 126, 130, 135, 149, 195, 197

Amphetamine Dependence, 101, 149

Antidotes, 128

B

Baclofen, 12, 19, 52, 197

Behavioral Addiction, 2, 11, 13, 17, 72, 88, 90-91, 93, 157, 160

Behavioral Therapy, 10-11, 18, 58, 61, 81, 88, 93, 106, 124, 148, 160, 165, 183, 188

Behavioral Treatments, 61

Behavioural Manifestations, 93

Biomolecular Mechanisms, 6, 60, 85, 90

Biosynthesis, 29-30

Blood Tests, 32, 44

Body Fluids, 30, 70

Borderline Personality Disorder, 35, 87, 117

Buprenorphine, 107, 145-147, 150, 178-179, 183-184, 197, 206

C

Cannabinoid Addiction, 12

Central Nervous System, 26, 34, 36, 52, 55, 169

Cocaine Addiction, 2, 18, 100, 117, 120, 124

Cocaine Dependence, 17-19, 142, 172, 208

Compulsion, 2, 15, 90, 130, 187

Contraindications, 55, 169, 176

D

Detoxification, 32, 45, 51, 105, 141, 147, 158, 167, 180-181, 183, 194-195

Diamorphine, 146-147

Dopamine, 2, 6, 8, 11, 20, 27, 36, 44, 47, 52-55, 58-67, 73-74, 79, 85, 91-92, 122-124, 132, 135, 141, 149, 156, 161-162, 172, 206

Dopamine Receptor Pathways, 122

Drug Misuse, 103, 130, 150, 196

Drug Overdose, 124, 128-129, 138, 148, 180

Dual Addictions, 47

E

Endogenous Compounds, 67

F

Food Addiction, 2-3, 14, 17, 72-74, 76

Functional Groups, 70, 122

G

Gambling Addiction, 2-3, 10, 76, 78, 91

Gender Difference, 38

Genetic Predisposition Testing, 44

Glutamate, 7-9, 13, 36, 47, 52, 59, 64, 66, 156, 169-170

Group Counseling, 159

Group Therapy, 32, 45, 99, 138, 158

Guardianship, 99

H

Heroin-assisted Treatment, 147

I

Immigrants, 51, 114, 150

Impulsivity, 54, 95, 105-106, 142, 162

In-person Support Groups, 88

L

Long-term Residential, 158

M
Medical Classifications, 84, 91
Mesocorticolimbic Pathway, 6-7
Mesolimbic Pathway, 3, 7, 27, 58, 64, 120, 178
Metabolic Pathways, 67
Methadone, 12, 104, 107, 138, 145-147, 149-150, 178-179, 183-184, 197, 209
Motivational Interviewing, 10, 82, 106, 183

N
Naltrexone, 11, 27, 32, 46-47, 107, 142, 147, 168-169, 173-181, 184, 221-222
Neuropsychology, 2
Neurotransmitters, 13, 26, 53, 59, 63, 66, 132, 170
Nicotine, 2, 5, 12-14, 17, 19-31, 60, 85, 90, 100, 104, 126, 132, 135, 153-154, 167, 183-184, 188, 198-206, 209, 222
Non-opioid Receptor Genes, 143
Norepinephrine, 27-28, 53, 62-65, 67, 78

O
Online Support Groups, 88, 189
Opioid Addiction, 12, 147, 175, 178-179, 206
Opioid Intoxication, 140, 175
Opioid Overdose, 126, 128, 138, 140-141, 144, 174, 176
Opioid Receptors, 47, 142, 176-177
Opioid Use Disorder, 101, 138, 141, 143-144, 149, 179

P
Peer Support, 82, 138
Pharmacodynamics, 26, 63
Pharmacokinetics, 28, 66, 169, 178, 204, 207
Pharmacological Treatment, 98
Psychoactive Effects, 19-20, 26, 31
Psychological Mechanisms, 80
Psychosis, 17, 48, 53, 56-58, 62, 105, 107, 116, 142, 194-195, 197
Psychostimulant Addiction, 11-12, 124
Public Health Definitions, 101

R
Racemic Amphetamine, 53, 68-70, 72
Recovery Programs, 87, 185
Refugees, 114, 150
Reinforcement Disorders, 24
Relationship Counselling, 87
Reward Sensitization, 1, 5, 8-9, 14, 60

S
Self-help, 45, 82, 89, 99, 106, 193, 219
Self-registration Techniques, 99
Serotonin, 20, 47, 58, 64-65, 73, 75, 78, 98-99
Sexual Addiction, 2, 14, 17, 84-90
Shopping Addiction, 3, 17, 93-99
Social Barriers, 43
Step-based Programs, 81
Street Children, 114
Substance Abuse, 4, 13, 15, 79, 100-101, 114-117, 130-131, 150, 153, 155, 157, 161-165, 191, 194, 196-200, 208, 210, 214, 218-219, 221
Substance Use Disorder, 9, 54, 101, 106-107, 115-116, 130, 137-138, 141-142, 148-149, 160, 191, 195, 197-198, 220
Substance-induced Disorders, 116
Substance-related Disorder, 101, 115
Substituted Derivatives, 69
Suicide Rates, 79-80
Sympathetic Nervous System, 27

T
Topiramate, 11, 19, 52, 184
Toxicity, 24-25, 51, 62, 126, 143, 146, 176
Transgenerational Epigenetic Inheritance, 5

V
Value Judgment, 104

W
Withdrawal Symptoms, 10-11, 17-18, 24, 36-37, 41, 52, 61, 72-73, 92, 102-103, 106-107, 116, 130-133, 135, 139, 142, 146, 158